The Stuntwoman's Workout

Library of Congress Cataloging in Publication Number: 20004111902

ISBN: 1-59474-030-5

Printed in Singapore

Typeset in Conduit, Garamond

Designed by Michael Rogalski

Photography by Damian Achilles

Distributed in North America by Chronicle Books
85 Second Street
San Francisco, CA 94105

10 9 8 7 6 5 4 3 2 1

Quirk Books
215 Church Street
Philadelphia, PA 19106
www.quirkbooks.com

Photo credits: pp. 5, 11, 15, 77, 190, courtesy of Heineken;
pp. 12, 96–97, 144–45, 186–88, courtesy of Sony Pictures Television;
pp. 115, 159, photos by Jim Abel.

The Stuntwoman's Workout

*Get Your Body
Ready
for Anything*

By **Danielle Burgio**

with Jennifer Worick

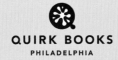

QUIRK BOOKS
PHILADELPHIA

To the entire stunt community,
whose dedication and energetic view of life
are the foundation of this book.
Thanks for welcoming me into your prestigious circle
and encouraging me to become more daring,
on set and off.

Table of Contents

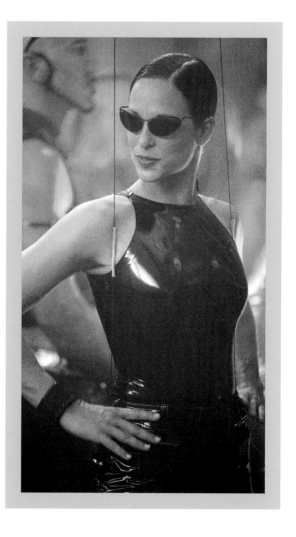

Wherever you go,
go with all your heart.
—Confucius (551BC–479BC)

Pleasure and action make
the hours seem short.
—William Shakespeare (1564–1616)

Foreword

I first met Danielle Burgio in New Mexico on the set of my movie *Vampires*. My stunt coordinator, Jeff Imada, hired her to portray the first vampire to attack our intrepid band of heroes as they explore an abandoned farmhouse in the opening of the film.

When it came time for the first attack, I yelled "action," and suddenly Danielle came hurtling in out of nowhere, air rammed from the shadows, ripping and clawing and growling and hissing and generally causing much mayhem until she was finally dispatched by a good, healthy dose of sunlight. After the first take, I was delighted. Danielle was fantastic.

It isn't simply that Danielle impresses as a talented stunt performer; she is also a talented actress in her own right. Stunt performer. Dancer. Athlete. Actress. Danielle is one of the best I've worked with.

And now you're reading her book, *The Stuntwoman's Workout*. So enjoy. And good luck with the workout. Make no mistake, this is the real deal here. If you master some of these exercises, you'll be ready for anything.

And if a bit of Danielle's excitement for life rubs off on you, all the better. Just remember her motto: "It's easy to master a skill when you are passionate about it."

John Carpenter
Los Angeles

Introduction
Go Big or Go Home!

When people first find out that I'm a stuntwoman, they want to know two things:

What do I do to work out?

And, what do I do for fun?

These sound like simple questions, but for me they are not so cut and dried. My answer provides the inspiration for this book:

My workout is my fun and my fun is my workout.

There are so many misconceptions about fitness, and often the idea of having to work out leads to resentment. I'm here to tell you that there is an awful lot of happiness in a little bit of physicality if you approach it the right way. I intend to transform your conception of working out into fun. If you aren't having fun, then you simply haven't found what works for you. I want you to find the workout that seems like a treat every time you do it.

Through my work, I've found many new activities to keep me engaged. Because each stunt requires different skills, I have discovered the benefits of the lessons I will be sharing with you in the following chapters.

It's important to stay strong. The body is an instrument that needs to be kept as tuned-up as possible, especially for an extreme situation. When getting bashed around is just another day at the office, I'd better be strong and resilient, with muscles that can pad and protect my body. And I need agility and physical aptitude to adapt to every situation.

It's important to stay grounded. On set, my Number 1 goal is to eliminate the danger and the possibility for injury. It takes a tremendous amount of focus to prepare for unforeseen circumstances. With actors, equipment, and explosions all around, a lot can go wrong if I'm not focused. It's imperative that I am physically and mentally stable. The greatest stunt people are talented athletes with good heads on their shoulders—and they all *love* what they do.

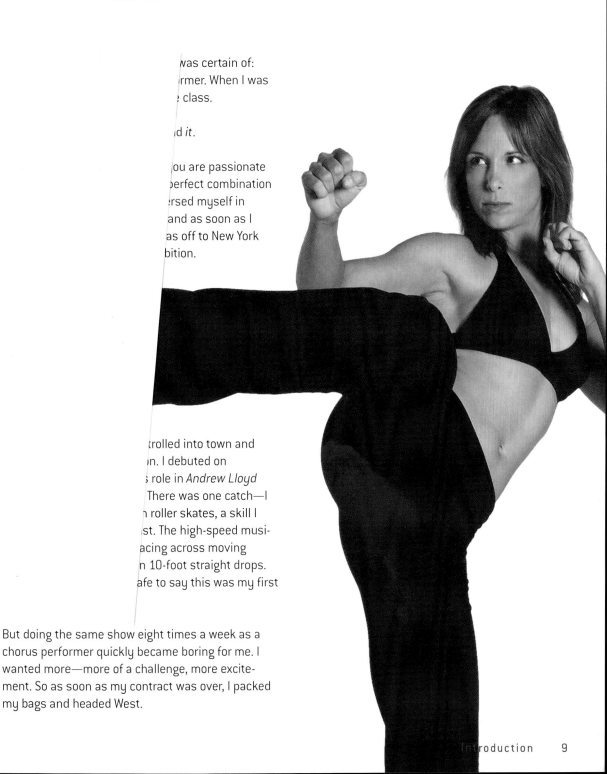

was certain of:
rmer. When I was
class.

d *it*.

ou are passionate
perfect combination
rsed myself in
and as soon as I
as off to New York
bition.

trolled into town and
n. I debuted on
role in *Andrew Lloyd*
There was one catch—I
roller skates, a skill I
st. The high-speed musi-
acing across moving
10-foot straight drops.
afe to say this was my first

But doing the same show eight times a week as a
chorus performer quickly became boring for me. I
wanted more—more of a challenge, more excitement. So as soon as my contract was over, I packed
my bags and headed West.

Finding My Calling

When I first got to Los Angeles, I thought I would put my dancing behind me and quickly transition into becoming a leading lady. As if it were that easy! Even though I was dying to break away from my old career, dancing paid the bills and, at least in Hollywood, it meant getting more film, television, and commercial work.

Through that work, I met some stuntpeople. At that time, my soul was open for a change. The timing was good. I watched the stuntpeople on set and thought, "I'm an athlete. I can do that." And before I knew it, by being in the right place at the right time (and through a bit of luck), I ended up on the set of *John Carpenter's Vampires*.

It began when, out of the blue, I received a call from Hollywood stunt legend Jeff Imada (*The Bourne Supremacy*, *Daredevil*, *The Crow*). I was honest. I told him I was totally green and didn't know if I would be able to handle the job. But Jeff said he loved working with dancers, because they understand body mechanics, are flexible, and are great at retaining choreography. He convinced me it would be easy for me to pick up.

I fell for it.

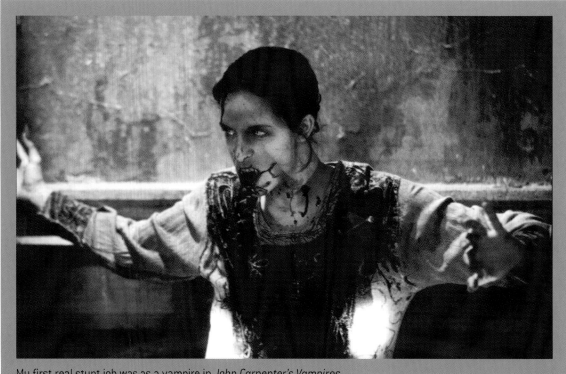

My first real stunt job was as a vampire in *John Carpenter's Vampires*.

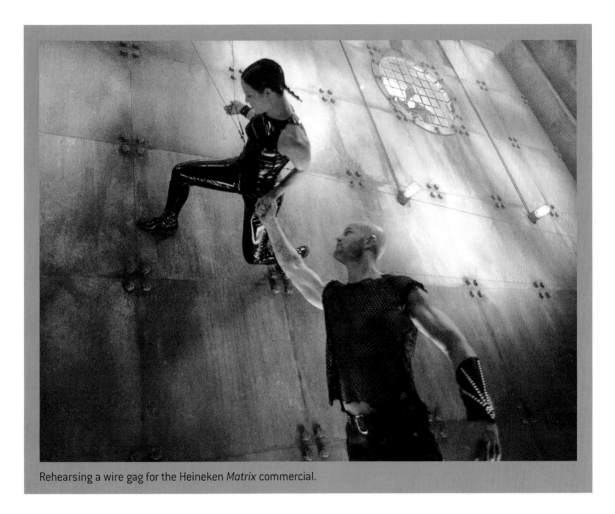

Rehearsing a wire gag for the Heineken *Matrix* commercial.

I arrived on set and was immediately thrown into doing full-blown, hardcore stunts. I got a literal crash course! I learned about air rams, ratchets, and squibs. I flew, I fought, I fell. Everything was blowing up around me, and I came off that movie on a total high. With 1,000 bruises and some blood loss, I came out of battle completely battered . . . and I was ecstatic.

I was reeling for months. It was so much fun! I completely shifted gears, quit my dance/acting agency and classes, and declared that I was going to be a stuntwoman. Based on the skills I already had, I thought it best to focus on martial arts and gymnastics, so I took classes and dove in.

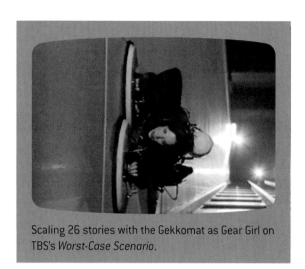

Scaling 26 stories with the Gekkomat as Gear Girl on TBS's *Worst-Case Scenario*.

Veteran stuntpeople say, "Go big or go home." I went big! I trained hard core five days a week and whipped my body into the best shape it's ever been. Everything in my life just clicked. Things started happening. More important, I let them. I was instantly in the elite stunt circle and rising to the top quickly. In 2001, after working on various movies, I ended up stunt doubling for Carrie-Anne Moss in *The Matrix Reloaded* and *The Matrix Revolutions*. I realized that I had hit the big time. What was going to top this?

Less than halfway through filming, I got a call to co-host *Worst-Case Scenario*, a new television series for TBS Superstation. The scheduling seemed impossible to work out, but through perseverance, I was able to have my cake and eat it too. Being Trinity's double turned out to be a dream job, and as "Gear Girl" on *Worst-Case*, I had a wonderful opportunity to train in skydiving, scuba diving, and paragliding, among other extreme skills. Best of all, I got my first taste of the media exposure that comes with being on a new series. That path led me to write this book, and it has given me the chance to share with you my knowledge and passion.

Here's the one big thing I've learned through all these experiences: Adventure is right around the corner if you simply open yourself up to it. That lesson is one of the key themes of this book.

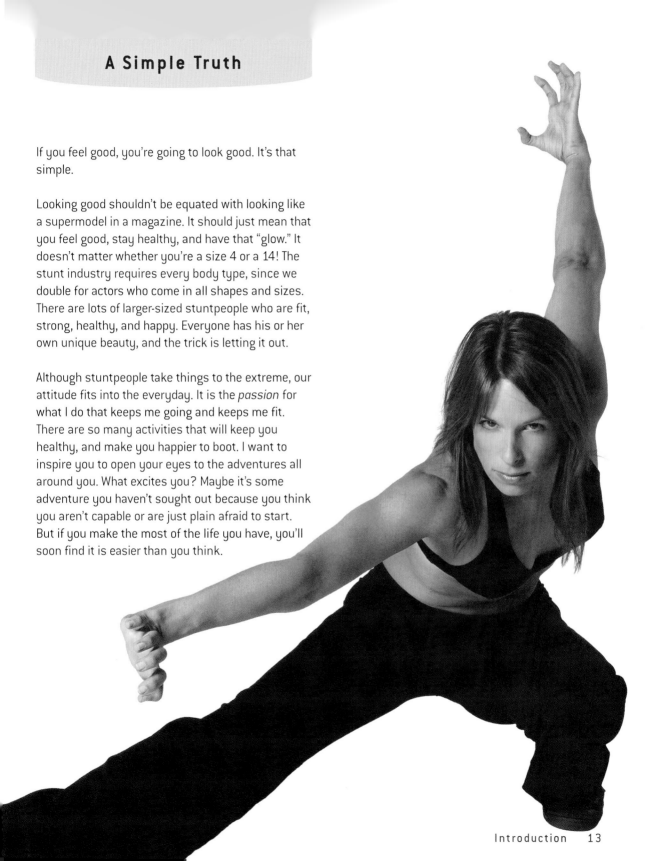

A Simple Truth

If you feel good, you're going to look good. It's that simple.

Looking good shouldn't be equated with looking like a supermodel in a magazine. It should just mean that you feel good, stay healthy, and have that "glow." It doesn't matter whether you're a size 4 or a 14! The stunt industry requires every body type, since we double for actors who come in all shapes and sizes. There are lots of larger-sized stuntpeople who are fit, strong, healthy, and happy. Everyone has his or her own unique beauty, and the trick is letting it out.

Although stuntpeople take things to the extreme, our attitude fits into the everyday. It is the *passion* for what I do that keeps me going and keeps me fit. There are so many activities that will keep you healthy, and make you happier to boot. I want to inspire you to open your eyes to the adventures all around you. What excites you? Maybe it's some adventure you haven't sought out because you think you aren't capable or are just plain afraid to start. But if you make the most of the life you have, you'll soon find it is easier than you think.

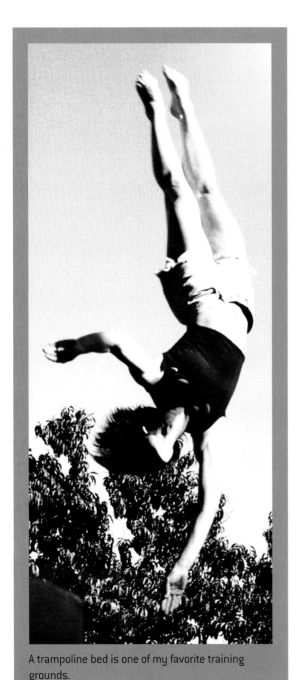

A trampoline bed is one of my favorite training grounds.

Working out at the gym is good for releasing endorphins, getting your heart rate up, and fitting some physical activity into your crowded schedule, but this book isn't about treadmills and elliptical trainers. It's about climbing a rock or riding a wave. It's about feeling like you're giving yourself a treat and addressing your mind, body, and spirit. The health benefits are the *consequence* of doing stuff that makes you happy.

We all have control over what our lives are and will be. And it's never too late to take action! So why not choose to get the most out of life and live the adventure, because there's so much out there to be had.

In the pages that follow, I am going to share with you some of my favorite exercises and activities that I have learned from some truly wonderful athletes and teachers. I've also included complete warm-up and cool-down routines that you can easily incorporate into your daily life. Along the way, you'll learn my secrets as a successful and deliriously happy stuntwoman, from what I keep in my medicine cabinet to how I stay motivated at the gym.

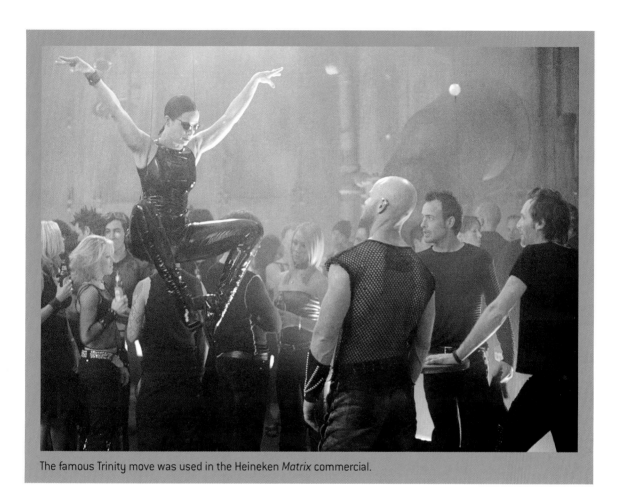

The famous Trinity move was used in the Heineken *Matrix* commercial.

But the most important thing I want you to do is choose to be active. There are hundreds of ways to adopt an overall active lifestyle. Go out hiking in the mornings and go dancing in the evenings. Take an active vacation—like skiing or snowboarding—instead of sitting on the beach. And even if you're at the beach, why not try rollerblading on the boardwalk or playing volleyball by the seaside? Going to Egypt? Climb the pyramids! Visiting France? Rent a bike while traveling around Cannes. Whatever your destination, explore as much as possible on foot. Opportunity for activity is all around you. Even something as simple as choosing to take the stairs rather than the elevator adds up to greater health and happiness over time.

Picking Your Passion

Now that you can't wait to climb a mountain (or even jump off of one), let's take the "work" out of "workout" and put some "act" into a kick-ass "activity." Here are just a few ideas to get you inspired. Most of these sports encompass all of these skills and muscle groups, but this chart highlights the main elements used in each sport.

	Legs	Back/Biceps	Chest/Triceps/Shoulders	Abs	Endurance	Focus	Flexibility	Coordination	Speed
BASE-jumping,* skydiving*						•			
Baseball, softball	•		•		•	•		•	•
Basketball	•				•	•		•	•
Biking—BMX	•	•	•	•	•	•		•	•
Biking—motocross*	•	•	•	•	•	•		•	•
Biking—mountain	•				•			•	
Bowling	•					•	•		
Boxing*	•	•		•	•	•			•
Broadsword			•			•		•	
Cycling	•				•				•
Dancing	•			•	•		•	•	
Fencing	•					•		•	
Football, rugby	•	•	•	•	•	•		•	•
Golf						•			
Gymnastics	•	•	•	•	•	•	•	•	•
Hang-gliding, Paragliding*								•	
Hiking	•				•				
Hockey	•	•	•	•	•	•		•	•

	Legs	Back/Biceps	Chest/Triceps/Shoulders	Abs	Endurance	Focus	Flexibility	Coordination	Speed
Martial arts—hard styles*	•	•	•	•	•	•	•	•	•
Martial arts—soft styles						•	•	•	
Racquet sports—squash, racquetball, tennis	•		•		•	•		•	•
Rafting,* kayaking, canoeing		•	•			•			
Rock climbing*	•	•		•	•	•	•	•	
Running	•				•				•
Skating—quads, inline, ice	•				•			•	
Skiing—downhill;*snowboarding*	•							•	
Skiing—cross-country	•	•			•				
Surfing*	•		•			•		•	
Swimming	•	•	•	•				•	
Trampoline				•	•			•	
Volleyball	•					•	•	•	
Water-skiing, Wakeboarding*	•	•	•			•		•	•
Wrestling	•	•	•	•	•	•	•	•	•
Yoga	•	•	•	•		•	•		

* adrenalin rush!

First Things First

Warm up, warm up, warm up. I can't say it enough. It is tremendously important to begin with a solid warm-up no matter what activity you are about to engage in. In this section I am going to teach you a quick and easy warm-up that will prime your entire body. If you are embarking on an activity that you know is going to put extra stress on a particular muscle (like your calves, for example, if you plan on running), spend some extra time warming up that muscle group.

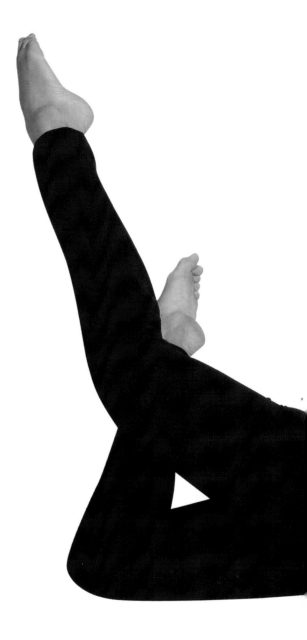

Warming up is most important when you're learning new skills. Anytime you introduce something new to your body, you encounter muscles you never knew you had. As a result, those muscles are going to be sore—and ultimately, that's a good thing. You want to know that you're making progress, making your muscles stronger. However, you don't want them so sore that you need to use your arms just to get your leg on the gas pedal. I can't tell you how many times I've had to do just that. I have hundreds of memories of waking up, putting my feet on the floor, and feeling pain shoot through my body just with the effort of trying to stand. And so I give to you my best advice. Yes, you got it—warm up!

The *Matrix* sequels are the first examples that come to mind when I think of the tremendous physical exertion that actors and stuntpeople put themselves through on a daily basis. Each one of us underwent months of training: several hours every day of pushing the body to its limits. Even for the simplest move in a fight scene—for example, reacting to a punch—it was extremely important to warm up the neck by doing head rolls. Otherwise, you were liable to wake up the next day feeling like you had whiplash.

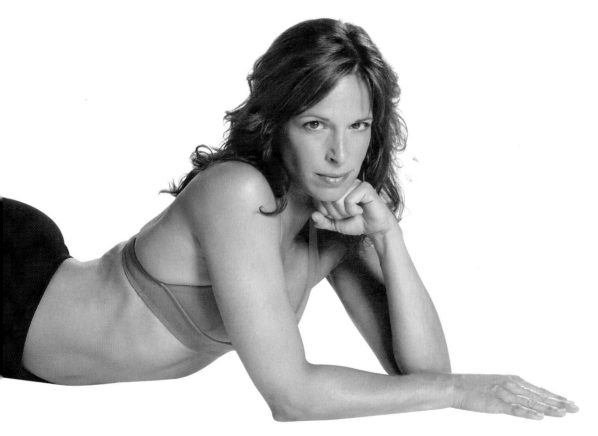

Heat and Ice

If you find yourself in an extreme situation, as I often do, I recommend heat and ice to help warm or cool your muscles. A hot bath or Jacuzzi is excellent therapy for sore muscles. And when you've pushed too hard to the point where you've strained yourself, ice is the answer. On the *Matrix* set, it was fairly common for the performers to end the day in a tub of ice. Any one of the cast members could tell you how unpleasant yet therapeutic an ice bath is.

Here's a good general rule for injuries. It's called the RICE method, which stands for Rest, Ice, Compress, Elevate. Use this guideline 24 to 72 hours after you've hurt yourself. For the first couple of days, lay off the injury. Keep it lightly wrapped and, as often as you can, make sure to raise it above your heart level to keep the blood from rushing to it. And don't forget the ice: The general rule is 20 minutes on and 40 minutes off to keep the swelling down. After the 72 hours, you can combine ice and heat therapy by using the following technique: 20 minutes of ice, 40 minutes of rest, 20 minutes of heat, 40 minutes of rest. Repeat as many times as possible—the longer, the better.

Tip:
A bag of frozen peas makes an awesome ice pack!

Any day that wasn't on camera was spent in the training hall (an airline hangar set up as a gym), stretching, practicing martial arts skills, doing cardio exercises, pumping iron, and basically doing whatever we could to keep our bodies strong and flexible. I would stretch in the morning when my body was locked up from the day before, continue stretching throughout the day to keep myself going, and then I'd stretch again as a cool-down. When people find out what I did on the set, some invariably quip, "Tough job to be able to work out all day." And my reply is always that it was the greatest job of my life . . . and the toughest.

The cool-down process is just as important as your warm-up. Do the same routine at the end of your workout, again paying special attention to the muscles you've worked the hardest. Believe me, you'll thank yourself the next morning. Your muscles will usually wait a day or even two to let you know that they are sore, so be good to them after you've worked them.

One last thing about warming up and cooling down: I want you to get in the habit of *paying attention to your body*. It will talk to you if you are willing to listen, giving you feedback about problem areas that might be too tight or especially tender. Your stretching routine is an excellent time to turn your focus to yourself and get connected. Once you and your body start communicating, you will start to see some amazing results.

The Stuntwoman's Medicine Cabinet

Here are my personal favorites: the staples of my medicine cabinet and stunt bag.

- **Antibiotic ointment**
  It's great for protecting wounds as well as helping the healing process. Make sure you clean the wound before application.

- **Arnica**
  Great for bruising and soreness, arnica improves circulation and comes in pill, gel, cream, and oil forms. For muscle soreness after a hard workout, take it orally. If you hit yourself and know there is a bruise forming, take it orally. If you already have a full-blown bruise, use it topically (I prefer the oil). Taking it both ways is not going to hurt you.

- **Biofreeze**
  An anti-inflammatory gel that works like ice for anything that's swollen. It also has a soothing analgesic effect.

- **Chinese remedies**
  Dit da jow is a liquid antiseptic that's great for treating strains, sprains, swelling, and bruising. Ching Wan Hung is a soothing balm I use for burns.

- **Emergen-C packets**
  A powder packet that is high in Vitamin C and electrolytes. I love to pop it into my water bottle before working out.

- **Gauze and saline**
  For cleaning wounds.

- **Hydrogen peroxide**
  For killing bacteria.

- **Ibuprofen**
  I take this only as an anti-inflammatory; never take it to get through a workout. Masking the pain only does additional damage.

- **Sea/Epsom salts**
  Add to the bath to relax and de-stress.

- **Sunscreen**
  Protects against the extra wear and tear on your skin when exercising outdoors.

- **Tegaderm**
  A true favorite of mine, Tegaderm is a bandage that seals a wound and allows the body to quickly heal itself. I have found it to be the best preventive against scarring. It is available over the counter, but you might have to ask the pharmacist for it.

- **Vitamins/Minerals**
  I take a multivitamin with one meal every day.

Warm-up and Cool-down Exercises

During this entire warm-up, try to keep your movement fluid. One motion should flow into the next so that you are never stopping your momentum and energy. Do these exercises at your own pace as you move from one body part to the next.

Roll It Out

Before you even begin to stretch, warm your body with this rolling technique to get your blood flowing.

❶ The key to this exercise is to keep your body loose. Stand with your feet slightly apart, arms by your sides.

❷ Start by gently dropping your head forward then rolling it in a circular motion toward your shoulders and back: first in a clockwise direction a few times, and then counterclockwise as well, taking note of any areas of stiffness or tenderness.

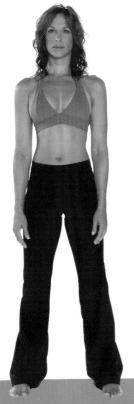

❶

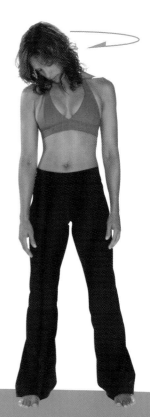

❷

❸ Now roll your shoulders, making a full backward circle that goes up toward your ears, back behind you, and then all the way back to your starting position. Do this roll a few times and then reverse it, making a forward circle several times.

❹ Repeat step 3, this time letting your arms follow your shoulders to create larger circles. You are beginning to generate more movement and more blood flow.

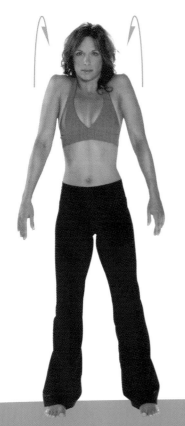

❸

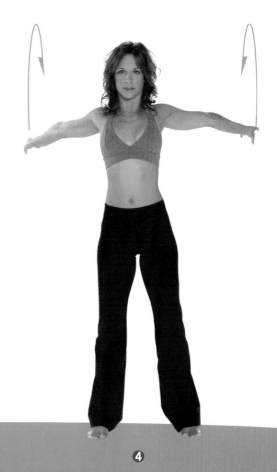

❹

❺ Now drop your arms and keep your body loose as you begin to make large circles with your torso. You'll do this roll without bending at the waist, with the circles originating from the ribcage. Circle clockwise a few times and then repeat in the opposite direction.

❻ Continue by making clockwise circles with your hips a few times and then reverse direction.

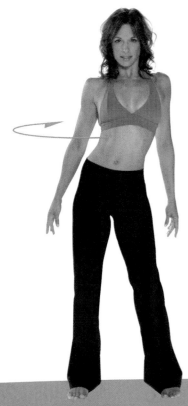

❺

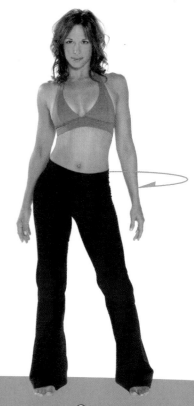

❻

❼ Shift your weight onto your left leg. With the ball of your right foot on the floor, make clockwise circles with your right knee. This will warm your hip joint, your knee, and your ankle. Reverse and make counterclockwise circles.

❽ Now shift your weight to your right leg and repeat step 7 with your left foot and knee.

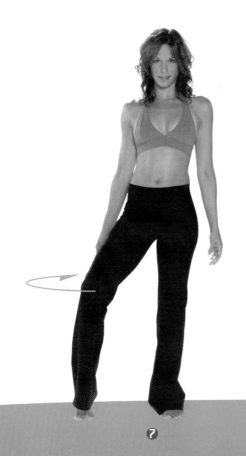

❼

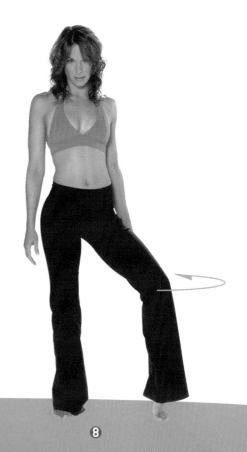

❽

Stretch 1

1. Place your feet hip-width apart and tuck your chin into your chest. Begin to roll your head, neck, and upper back forward and toward the ground, rolling your spine all the way down, vertebra by vertebra, without forcing. No bouncing either! Let your arms simply hang forward.

❷ Relax and let your body weight hang so that you are now completely bent forward at the waist. You will feel a release in your lower back and a stretch in your hamstrings and glutes. Take a deep breath in and, on the exhale, allow yourself to sink deeper.

❸ Start bending at the knees and place your hands flat on the ground in front of your feet. Continue to squat, pushing your knees forward.

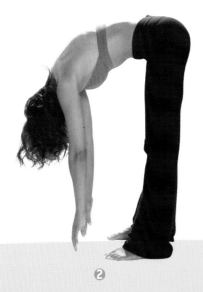

❷

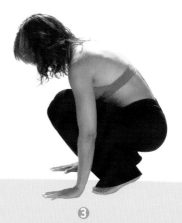

❸

④ Keeping your hands flat on the ground, rise up as high as you can on the balls of your feet to warm up your ankles and feet.

⑤ Push back, allowing your heels to return to the floor. As you straighten your legs, keep your chest as close to your thighs as possible.

6. Roll up slowly, one vertebra at a time.

7. Repeat steps 1 through 6 three times.

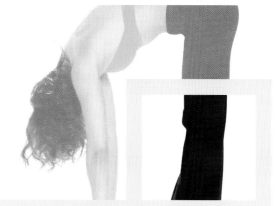

Focus on keeping your legs straight to increase the stretch in your hamstrings and glutes.

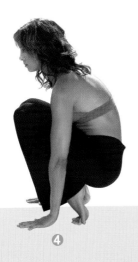

④

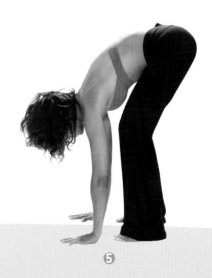

⑤

Warm-up and Cool-down Exercises

Stretch 2

1 Take a wider stance, this time with feet slightly outside of shoulder-width, toes pointed forward, and arms straight out to your sides.

2 Keep your body facing forward and your hips centered. Now, with your right arm reach, reach, reach up and over to your left as far as your body will allow without collapsing. You should maintain a strong, straight torso. Remember: no bouncing! You will feel the stretch along the entire right side of your torso.

3. Take a deep inhalation.

4. On the exhale, with your legs still facing forward, twist to the left from your waist, extending both arms out to your sides for balance. Bend at the waist, ideally 90 degrees to the floor, while keeping a flat back. You should feel the stretch going down the lower back, into the glutes, and into the hamstrings.

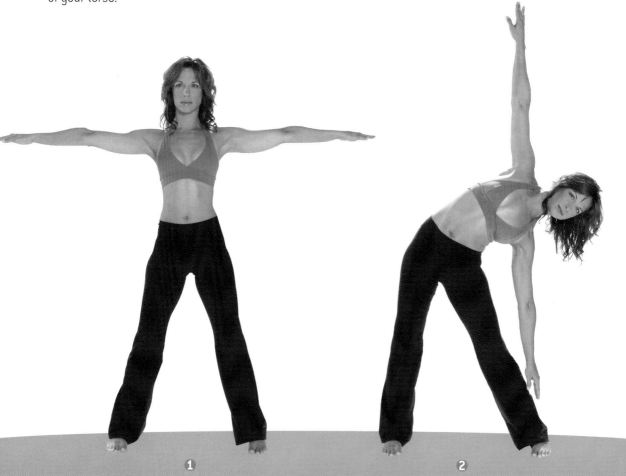

1 **2**

5 Take another deep breath, and on the exhale, keeping straight legs, continue bending at the waist. As you drop, first reach your belly button to your left thigh, then your chest to your knee so that your torso remains elongated. Place your hands comfortably on the floor for balance. This will stretch your left hamstring and calf.

6 As you come up, let your right arm lead you as it reaches up and over, keeping a flat back. This will open you back to your starting position, facing forward.

7. Repeat steps 1 through 6, this time reaching to the right with your left arm.

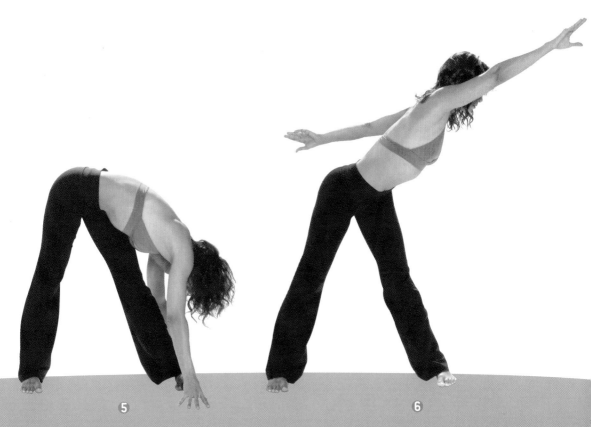

5

6

❶ Start with your feet slightly apart, arms by your sides.

❷ Bring your feet together and squat down, placing your hands on the floor in front of your knees for balance.

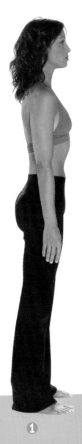

❶

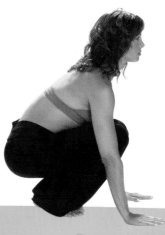

❷

③ Reach your right leg directly back as far as you can. Make sure your left knee is over your ankle and your toes are facing forward. Push your right heel toward the ground to increase the stretch in your right calf. Hold for several seconds.

④ Return your right foot to the squat position.

5. Repeat steps 2 through 4, this time with your left leg reaching back.

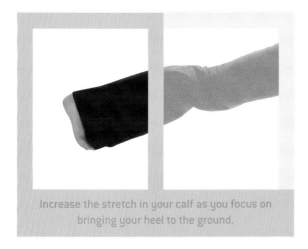

Increase the stretch in your calf as you focus on bringing your heel to the ground.

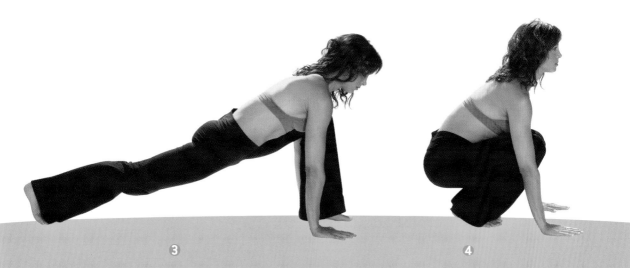

③   ④

❶ Sit on the floor with your legs folded underneath you. Your back should be straight and balanced.

❷ Keeping your knees on the floor, reach your arms behind you, fingers facing forward. Bend your elbows and feel the stretch in your quads and hip flexors.

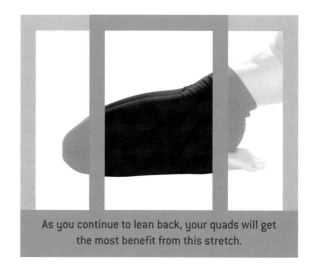

As you continue to lean back, your quads will get the most benefit from this stretch.

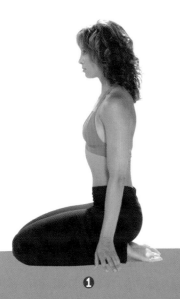

❶

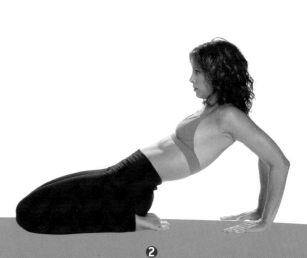

❷

3 Now, rotate your hands so your fingers are facing behind you. Slightly arch your back, press your shoulders blades together, lift your pelvis, and slowly drop your head back. This is a wonderful stretch for the entire front of your body.

4 Drop your pelvis and slowly and gently roll up to a straight sitting position. Your head should come up last. Keep your arms relaxed.

5. Repeat steps 1 through 4 three times. Increase the stretch with each rep.

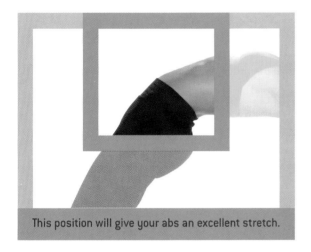

This position will give your abs an excellent stretch.

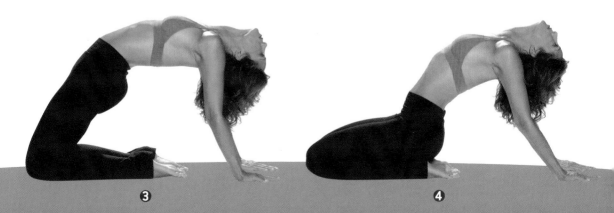

3

4

Chapter 1
Strength

Strength: *n.* the power to resist strain, stress, etc.; toughness; durability

There's a lot more to building strength than toning, sculpting, and beefing up your muscles. It's important to keep your body strong for many reasons that have nothing to do with mere appearance and size. The stronger you are, the healthier you are. Strong muscles make you more capable of any physical task you set out to do and less prone to injury. As you'll hear me say again and again, my goal is to get you to be strong, healthy, and happy. It's irrelevant whether you are a size 4 or size 14.

We all have different genetic dispositions. Some people are naturally muscular and simply don't have to work as hard as others. (We hate them!) No two bodies or psyches are exactly alike. It's up to you to find what works and feels right for you.

In the stunt world, all sorts of actresses need to be doubled. And from Calista Flockhart to Queen Latifah and all body types in between, all of their stunt-women have one thing in common: They are agile and strong.

In the film industry these days, women are on screen kicking ass more and more—in less and less clothing. Yes, sexy and revealing outfits are in. I admit that they look great on camera, and what person with a great body wouldn't want to get all decked out in some tight, skimpy leather? Well, that's all fine with me until they ask me to hurl my body down a flight of stairs! My solution? Build more muscle. Muscle tissue is an amazing substance that our bodies produce to provide excellent protection from injury.

When doubling for Jennifer Garner (Elektra) during a key rooftop fight sequence for *Daredevil*, my body was hurled into all kinds of nasty things. Now if you recall Elektra's tight-fitting, skimpy outfit, you'll understand why there was no room for the protective padding that I would normally put under my wardrobe. That sexy but evil Bullseye (Colin Farrell) threw me into several air ducts (metal corners are not very forgiving), onto the ground, and off the roof to a ledge that was coated with a gravel-like surface. I was left with some wicked road rash. My only saving grace was that I was smart enough to take the extra precaution to build some muscle mass ahead of time. And so I walked away with a few small battle scars but no broken bones.

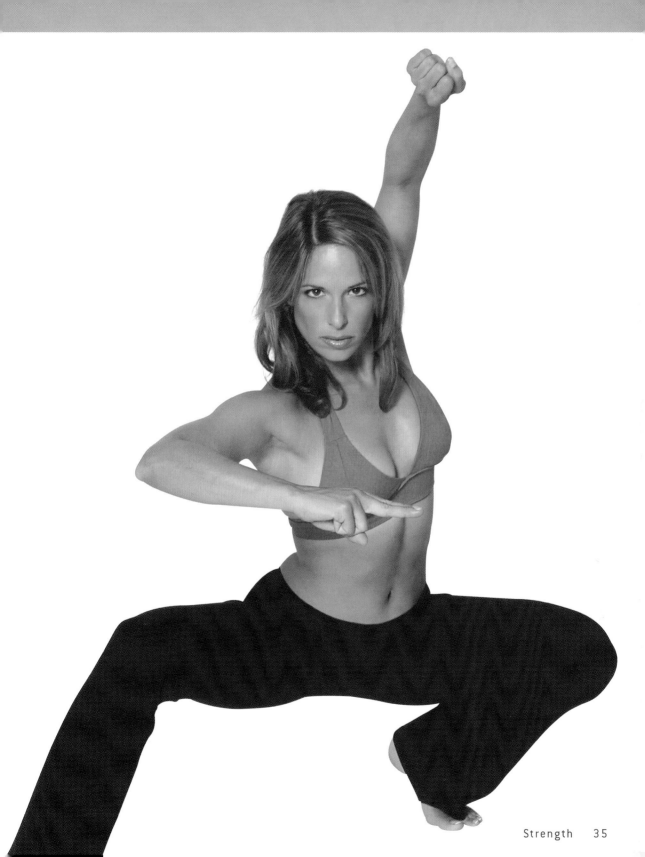

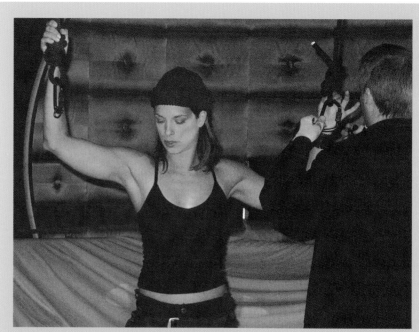

Getting harnessed and checking the rig for safety for one of my more common feats, an aerial flip.

Equally as important as having good muscle mass in my line of work is the benefit of strength itself. Too many times I recall saying to myself, *"Omigod, I hope I don't have to do another take because I don't know if my muscles will hold out any longer!"* During the freeway scene in *The Matrix Reloaded*, we needed to get a shot that would make it appear like Trinity (Carrie-Anne Moss) was jumping from an overpass onto a speeding motorcycle carrier. For the last part of the sequence, the directors wanted a close-up of the landing onto the bike carrier. Once the camera was set up behind the mounted motorcycles, we needed to find a way to make it look like I was dropping in from above. The solution was to set up a pull-up bar far enough above the camera shot so that I

could hoist my body up, hold myself out of the frame until the vehicle got up to speed, and then drop down. (All those chin-ups sure came in handy! The Classic Chin-ups/Pull-ups exercise is on pages 50–51.) Because of all the variables, it took several takes to get this scene right. By the end, I was wishing for my *own* stunt double, but my muscles came through for me in the end. Everybody was thrilled with the outcome, and it stands as one of my favorite sequences in the movie.

Word to the wise: Don't try this at home.

But what I *do* encourage you to do is to challenge yourself.

Setting Your Goals

The basic rules for strengthening depend on what kind of results you are looking for. In any of the following weight-training techniques, it's going to be up to you to determine the amount of weight to work with. I like the "pyramid technique": In doing three sets of repetitions, you gradually increase weight and decrease repetitions. There's a point where being really big doesn't mean you're really strong. Doing extremely low reps (for example, 6-4-2) focuses more on strength than size. Medium reps (12-10-8) are the most efficient way to build mass. High reps (20-plus) are best for toning. For any of these techniques, the most important rule is to push yourself to "failure." If you've set out to do 15 reps, then your fifteenth rep should be nearly impossible. If two is your goal, your second rep should be nearly impossible. Get the picture?

One other note: Your resting time between sets should be about one minute, which will allow your muscles to recover about 75 percent. If you rest too long, your muscles recover almost fully, which keeps you from using the additional muscle fibers needed to completely tax the muscle. Not enough rest taxes you cardiovascularly, which is not optimal for strength training.

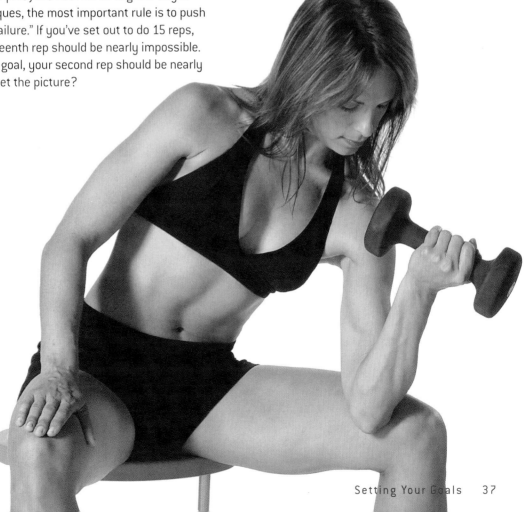

There is something to gain by both the "positive" (lifting) and the "negative" (lowering) movements of these exercises. By lifting a weight, you utilize one set of muscles; when you lower a weight, you use another set. Be sure to lower the weight just as deliberately as you've lifted it, and do not let gravity do the work for you. Even when you're doing calisthenics, remember that you're using your body as the "weight," so you should apply the same rules of focus and deliberate movement.

An average day at "the office" for me: On wires against a green screen in Hawaii for a commercial shoot.

When strength training, remember the theory of polar opposites. The body is a little like a pulley system and needs to be balanced. If you want to build your chest, don't forget your back. If you're going for those six-pack abs, don't neglect your lower back. Biceps and triceps go together, as do quadriceps and hamstrings. Got it?

You'll hear a lot of people preach about the benefits of low-impact exercise (elliptical trainer workouts and yoga, for example). However, there are also benefits to high-impact sports such as running and football. Basically, anything jarring to the body is considered *impact*. Your body is designed to adapt to its environment. The more impact you have, the denser and therefore stronger your bones become. But remember: Always listen to your body. You're going to know what's working for you. Know when to push but also know when to stop.

For example, it's going to be up to you to determine the difference between good pain and bad pain. While you're working to make your body stronger, you will feel pain. You *should* feel pain. Exercise breaks down muscle fibers, which then grow back even stronger. These growing pains let you know that you're making progress.

The best way that I know to describe the "good pain" is to call it a burning sensation that you feel in the belly of your muscle. On the other hand, "bad pain" is when you feel sharp pains, especially anywhere near your joints. You also want to avoid any clicking sensations in your joints, which are usually the result of something being out of place and bones or cartilage rubbing against each other. In any of these "bad" scenarios, consult a doctor and/or modify your exercise to avoid these sensations. If you ignore them, you're going to prolong the injury and build up scar tissue.

I know that working out can seem like a chore to some, but in my opinion it's all about your mental approach. I want to challenge you to find activities that you are interested in and that you can get passionate about. And then, I would like for you to use these exercises to help you achieve your fitness goal. For example, if you love the outdoors, maybe rock climbing is something that would inspire you to get physical. If so, check the chart on pages 16–17 and see what muscles you're going to need to help you climb a rock like Tom Cruise in *Mission Impossible*. And use the activity that inspires you to stay strong, healthy, and active.

What follows are some great exercises to get you started, to get your body primed and ready to take on a whole new outlook on life. But don't stop here; let this springboard you into an entirely new healthy, happy existence.

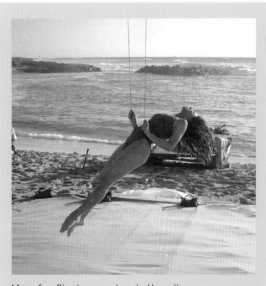

More fun flipping on wires in Hawaii.

Major Muscle Groups

Throughout the exercises that follow, you will be working these major muscle groups. Note that the more common names (shoulders, calves, glutes, abs, etc.) are used in the exercise instructions because, after all, not many of us use these anatomical terms.

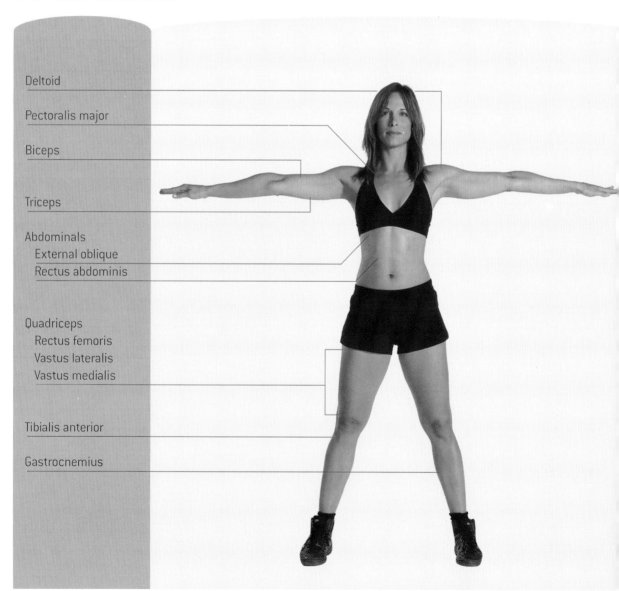

Deltoid

Pectoralis major

Biceps

Triceps

Abdominals
External oblique
Rectus abdominis

Quadriceps
Rectus femoris
Vastus lateralis
Vastus medialis

Tibialis anterior

Gastrocnemius

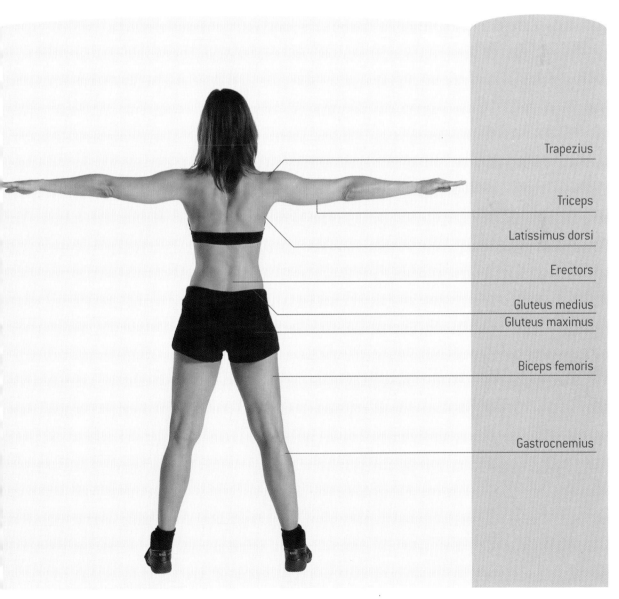

Trapezius

Triceps

Latissimus dorsi

Erectors

Gluteus medius
Gluteus maximus

Biceps femoris

Gastrocnemius

Strengthening Exercises

Now no cheating! You must do these exercises slowly and with proper form. The problem with doing things quickly is that inertia, rather than your actual muscle contraction, ends up moving the weight.

Remember that you want muscles to heal before you hit them up again; the bigger the muscle, the longer the recovery time (up to 3 days if you've really worked hard). Pick a day to do back and biceps, another day to do chest and triceps. Abdominal muscles heal really fast so they can be worked daily. (Sorry, but the truth hurts.) Start with the exercises that work the bigger muscles (quadriceps, back, chest) and work your way down until you are working the smaller muscles (calves, biceps, triceps). Keep in mind, however, that it's nearly impossible to isolate any one muscle; you almost always work several at a time.

The Perfect Form

All of these exercises have to start from good form. A simple standing position is not a resting position! Your body should be full of energy even while standing or in repose. Imagine a string at the crown of your head pulling you up so you have a straight line from the base of your spine through the top of your head, with your feet firmly planted into the ground. Make sure you maintain your form all the way through to the end of the exercise. If you cheat by being sloppy, you're only cheating yourself! If you practice the wrong thing repeatedly, you get really good at doing it wrong. Don't reinforce your own bad behavior.

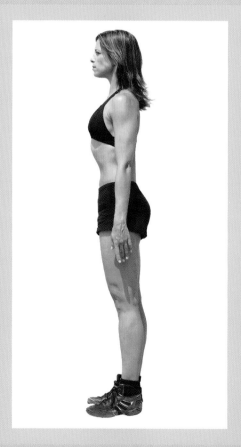

Note: For each of these exercises, the number of repetitions depends on your fitness level, the variations you've added, and the other exercises you are combining with this one. See the circuits at the end of the book for some combinations of exercises based on your fitness level.

I've included ratings next to each strengthening and speed exercise to denote the level of fitness the exercise is suited to. Of course, I want you to challenge yourself, so if you believe you are at level 2 but a level 4 exercise sounds intriguing, give it a go. But if it's a gymnastics trick and you're a beginner, do it with the assistance of an experienced spotter. Also keep in mind that, as a beginner, you may "work to failure" quickly at first (i.e., you will be able to do only a few reps initially).

Levels of fitness

Level 1: Beginner—starting from scratch.

Level 2: Slightly fit.

Level 3: Average level of fitness—does at least one sport regularly or hits the gym a couple of times a week.

Level 4: Passionate and consistent with one or more sport—stronger and more fit than the average bear.

Level 5: Phenomenal all-around athlete.

Strengthening rules

For each of the following exercises, there are three rules:

Rule 1: Warm up!

Rule 2: Use slow and controlled movement!

Rule 3: Go to failure!

Leg Strengthening

Oldie but Goodie Squats

Levels: 1–5

A squat is a compound movement that uses more than one muscle group: quads (thighs), lower back, and glutes (aka, the butt). It's great for building strength and mass. (Because these muscles are generally strong to begin with, it's ideal to add weights to get these muscles to work. See Variations, opposite page.)

① Stand tall with hands at your sides, keeping a straight back. Feet should be shoulder-width apart.

② Bend your knees, making sure your knees stay over your toes so you don't put any undue stress on your joints. Keep constant attention on the muscles you're working.

3. Slowly return to a standing position, keeping tension in the muscle.

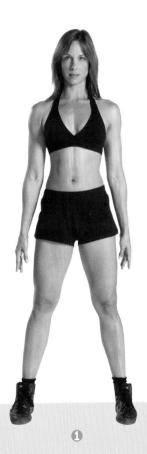

①

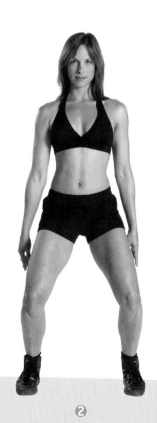

②

Variations:

- Widen your stance. Turn your legs out from the hips and bend your knees, remembering to keep your knees over your toes. This works the inner thighs.

- Keep your knees close together to work the outer thighs.

- Lean back against a wall and bend your knees until you are flat-backed against the wall with your legs at a 90-degree angle: Often referred to as "sissy squats," these are anything but!

- Add a platform: If you put your heels up on a platform even an inch high, you can take the strain off of your spinal erectors (lower back).

- Add hand weights, keeping your arms comfortably at your sides as you do each squat. It's up to you to pile on enough weight to take this exercise to failure, again depending on the results you want.

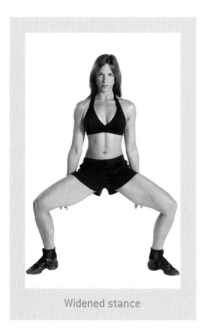

Widened stance

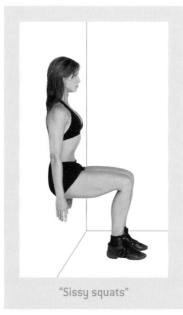

"Sissy squats"

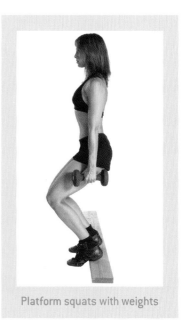

Platform squats with weights

Leg Strengthening

Basic Lunges

Levels: 1–5

This is a great exercise for legs, but it has the added benefit of working the glutes. Again, because these muscles are generally strong, adding hand weights is a great way to get these muscles to really work.

1. Stand tall, with your hands at your sides and your feet together. Keep a straight back.

❷ Step out with one foot, placing the heel down first and rolling your weight to the center of the foot. Always make sure the knees line up over the toes.

❸ Lower yourself until your front leg is bent at a 90-degree angle and your back knee touches the ground. Do not put any weight onto the back knee.

4. Slowly raise yourself, remembering to keep the weight on your heel.

5. Bring your feet together and repeat with your opposite leg.

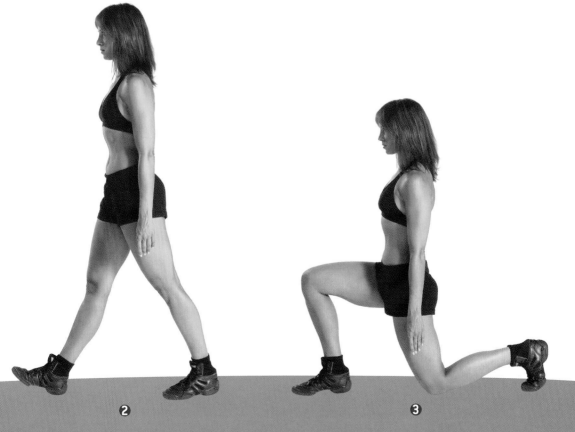

❷   ❸

Variations:

- Add a platform: By stepping onto a platform of some kind, you are engaging different leg muscles. The higher the platform, the harder the exercise.

- Add hand weights. Hand weights add resistance and make it harder to get up.

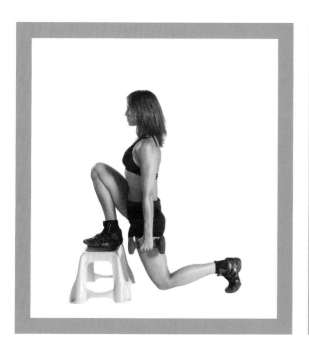 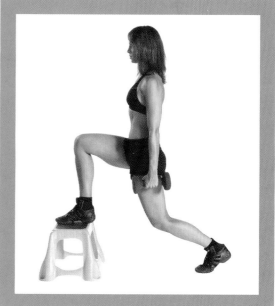

Leg Strengthening

Rise and Shine

Levels: 1–5

Known by dancers as relevés, these exercises specifically work the calves.

1. Start on any secured raised surface, such as a platform, curb, or stair, with the balls of your feet on the edge and your toes firmly on the platform. Keep straight legs and a straight back throughout this exercise.

❷ Lower your heels below the platform's edge.

❸ Raise your heels up so they're above the platform and you are standing on the balls of your feet.

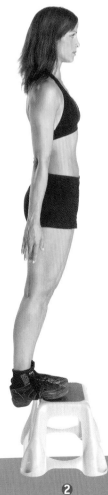

❷

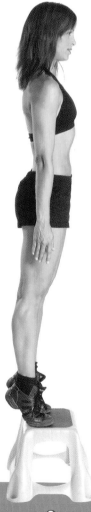

❸

Variations:

- To enhance this exercise, hold onto a rail for balance and do steps 1 through 3 with all of your weight on one foot. Next, switch to your opposite foot and repeat.

- Add hand weights to increase difficulty.

- If you don't have a platform, do this exercise flat from the ground and simply raise and lower your heels.

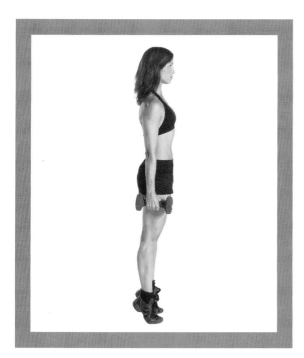

Weighing It Out

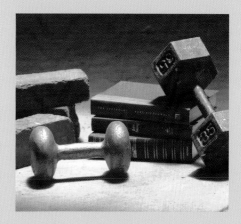

If you don't have weights on hand, improvise. Bricks, books, a bowling ball in a bowling bag, and even small children can all be used in lieu of dumbbells. And note that any weight that you hold onto will be a little extra pump for the forearm.

Swimming pools can act as a phenomenal training "ground"! Doing exercises in water supports your body while offering great resistance.

Back and Biceps Strengthening

Classic Chin-ups/Pull-ups

Levels: 4–5

They sound like very common exercises, but these are quite hard. You are pulling up the entire weight of your body. A chin-up is done with your palms facing away from you, while a pull-up is done with palms toward you. Both work the back and biceps, but a chin-up works the forearm more and is slightly more difficult. If you don't have access to a pull-up bar, you can substitute any horizontal bar that can bear your weight, such as a tree branch or exposed pipe. You can also purchase an inexpensive chin-up bar that can be installed in a doorframe.

1. Grab the bar at a comfortable arm width. The closer together the arms are, the more of the middle back you work and the easier the exercise is.

2. Pull your body up until your chin is higher than the bar. Bending your knees and crossing your ankles will help you stabilize your body.

3. Slowly lower your body until your arms are fully extended.

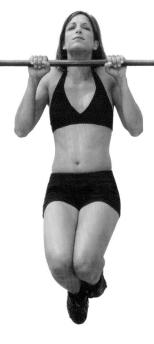

2

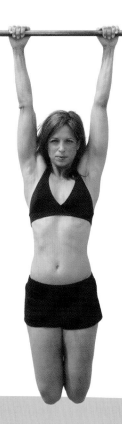

3

Variations:

- "Negatives" are an easier alternative. Step up on a chair under a pull-up bar, and get into position with your chin above the bar. Transfer the weight to your arms and take your feet off the chair by bending your knees. Lower your body slowly until you are hanging, arms fully extended. Step back onto the chair and repeat. This is a great way to work up to doing full-fledged pull-ups or chin-ups.

- Still easier, pull up with a partner: Grasp the bar, bend your knees, and have your partner cup your ankles. A little pressure from your partner's hands will make it easier for you to pull up. Don't be a sissy—do the work!

- Advanced version: With your hands in the chin-up position, pull up as hard as you can, getting your torso above the bar with your arms locked.

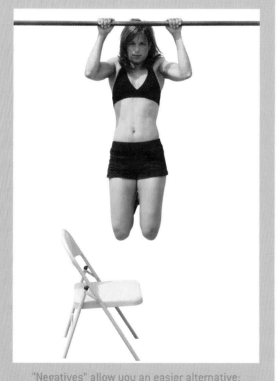

"Negatives" allow you an easier alternative: Use a chair to get in position above the bar.

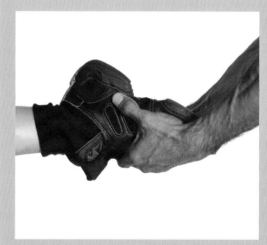

Have your partner cup your feet/ankles to give you added support on the chin-up or pull-up.

Back and Biceps Strengthening

Rope Climbs

Levels: 3–5

This is a great exercise once you've mastered your chin-ups. Sit-ups (page 64) and push-ups (page 56) are also excellent training for rope climbs. Back in the early 1900s, rope climbing was actually an Olympic event. It's still a great way to work your back (lats) and shoulders, and it's also amazing for building forearm and hand strength.

Find a thick rope, preferably one made of hemp and measuring 1½ inches (3.8 cm) in diameter. Using a double half hitch knot, hang the rope from something sturdy, such as a tree branch. Your body weight on the rope will cause the knot to tighten. For a little extra safety once the knot is tight, you can duct tape the loose end of the hanging rope.

When determining the length of rope you need, be sure to include extra length to accommodate your knot and leave a 5-foot (1.5 m) tail on the ground (you don't want the rope to flop around while you're climbing). In the beginning, the climbing won't be ideal. Ropes are much better once they are broken in. Serious rope climbers install a metal plate at the top of the rope so they have a goal to reach for. There's nothing like the sound of that tap to motivate you. Professionals are able to climb 20 feet (6 m).

This exercise can be murder on your hands, so professionals chalk the rope and chalk and tape their hands. Do what ya gotta do!

When starting out, get up the rope any way you can. A lot of beginners use their feet to help them shimmy up. Here's a good way to start:

1. Stand close to the rope and, as you reach up the length of the rope with your right arm, simultaneously kick up your left knee.

❷ As you reach with your left arm, kick your right knee up. You're using the kicking motion of your legs in opposition with your arms to give you momentum (just as you do when walking or running).

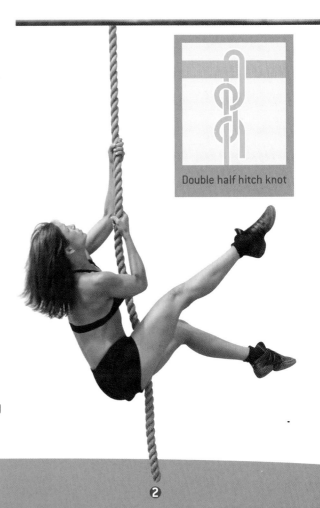

Double half hitch knot

❸ Lean back with a slight arch, driving your knees from side to side. Look up to see where you're going and gauge your progress.

Once you perfect this technique, try a little competition, like the pros do: Time your "personal best" climb from the ground to the plate.

Variation:

• This technique focuses more on pure strength, but you will be sacrificing your speed: Start in a seated position, with your legs out in front of you and the rope between your legs. As you climb, maintain your body in this L position for a much greater ab workout. You will often see circus performers assuming this position when working on ropes.

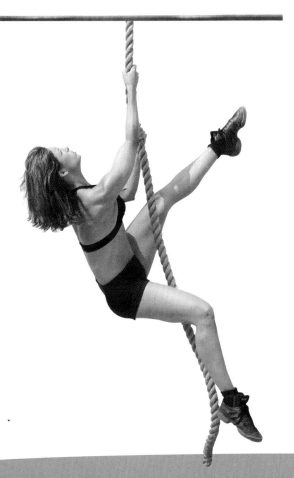

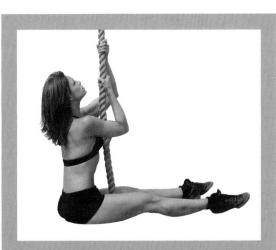

Beginning and maintaining an L position increases your abdominal workout.

❸

Back and Biceps Strengthening

The Bend and Stand

Levels: 1–5

This exercise is great for your lower back and your glutes. Because these muscles are generally strong, you are going to need to add weights to get these muscles to work.

❶ Start in a nice strong standing position, feet hip-width apart, arms straight and holding hand weights just in front of your thighs. (Once again, use the amount of weight that will allow you to "go to failure.")

2. Keeping a flat back and your head up, bend at the waist as far as you can, keeping strong, tight legs.

❸ Slowly return to standing position, squeezing your butt to lift your torso. Be careful not to overarch your back.

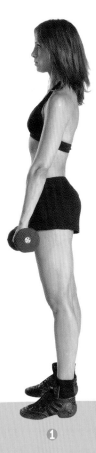

❶

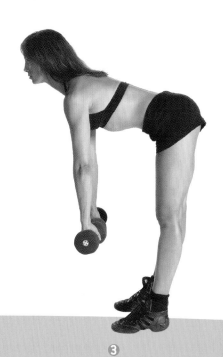

❸

Back and Biceps Strengthening

Bulging Bicep Curls

Levels: 1–5
This exercise isolates the biceps.

1 Grab yourself a hand weight. Sit on a chair or bench and place your right elbow on the inside of your right knee, with your arm straight.

2 As you bring the weight up, rotate your thumb away from you. At the top of the exercise, squeeze your bicep. This will help peak the muscle.

3. Slowly straighten your arm, rotating your wrist back to a straightened position. Do as many repetitions as you can with one arm and then switch arms and repeat.

Tip:
The reps and the weights will be determined by your level of expertise, but aim to do at least three sets on each arm.

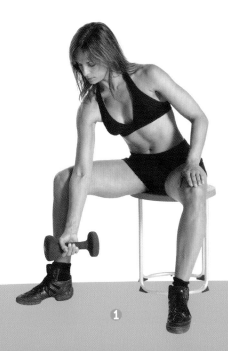

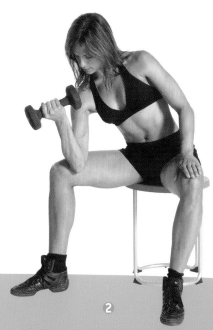

Chest, Shoulders, and Triceps Strengthening

Old School Push-ups

Levels: 2–5

In my opinion, push-ups are the single best overall exercise you can do. They work your shoulders, your chest, your triceps, and your abs. They are very challenging—and the best thing is, you can do them without props and in any location. When I'm working on a film and can't get to a gym, sit-ups and push-ups become my core exercises.

Note: I want to remind you to do these exercises *slowly* and with good form rather than just trying to crank them out and get them over with.

1. Lie facedown on the floor. Place your hands flat on the floor slightly outside of your shoulders. Fingers should point forward.

❷ With a flat back and straight legs, push up with your arms until they are fully extended. Keep your neck straight and don't let your chin drop.

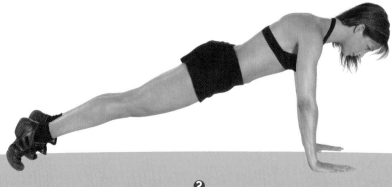

❷

❸ Slowly lower yourself as far as you can without touching the floor, again keeping your back, legs, and neck straight.

Tip:
Get a deck of cards. The card you flip is the amount of reps you do. Numbers are face value, face cards are 10, aces are 15, and jokers—far from lucky—are 20.

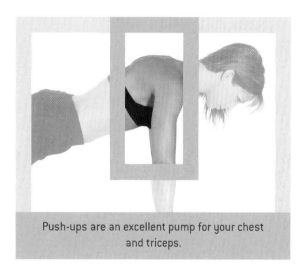

Push-ups are an excellent pump for your chest and triceps.

❸

Variations:

- Changing hand or elbow positions will allow you to work different parts of the chest and triceps. Experiment with different positions to see where you feel the burn. For example, either widen or close up the space between your arms, or rotate your fingers inward or outward.

- Add a weight to your back. Small children are great for this. (Seriously, I used to sit on my dad's back when he did his push-ups.)

- One-arm push-ups: The trick is to place your support hand on the ground directly beneath the center of your chest, rolling your opposite shoulder slightly back.

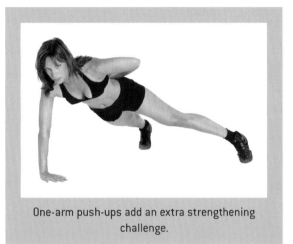

One-arm push-ups add an extra strengthening challenge.

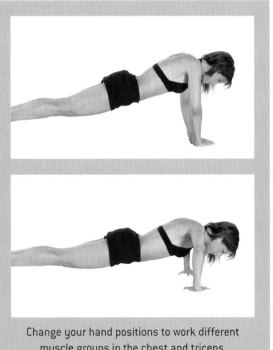

Change your hand positions to work different muscle groups in the chest and triceps.

Chest, Shoulders, and Triceps Strengthening

Handstand Push-ups

Levels: 3–5

You already know how much I love push-ups. This one is specifically designed to work your full shoulder. If you've never tried these before, realize that the wall is your friend: It will support you. If you're unsure about the exercise, you can always have a friend stand by your side for support and assistance.

1. Put your hands on the floor about a foot (0.3 m) away from a wall.

❷ Kick your legs up into a handstand, with your heels touching the wall.

3. Make sure to keep a straight back. Bend your elbows and lower your arms until your head is just above the ground.

4. Press back up and straighten your arms.

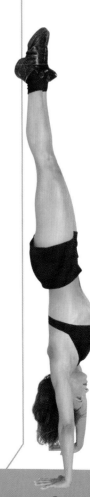

❷

Chest, Shoulders, and Triceps Strengthening

Handstand Snap Downs

Levels: 4–5

This is a favorite among gymnasts, since it helps develop the power needed to throw aerial tricks. For everyone else not striving for Olympic gold, it's a challenging but fun way to work the shoulders, triceps, and abs.

❶ This exercise starts from a handstand. If you need to learn this trick, practice against a wall or have a friend spot you by holding your ankles. But when you do the actual exercise, you will need to be clear of walls and obstacles. Make sure you are on a soft surface, such as grass or a mat.

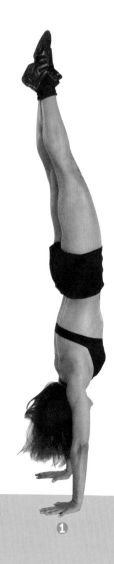

❶

❷ From a good handstand position, keeping your body strong and tight, simultaneously pop your hands off the floor and snap your feet under you, keeping your legs together.

❸ As your feet are coming down, your upper body snaps up, with your arms reaching toward the ceiling.

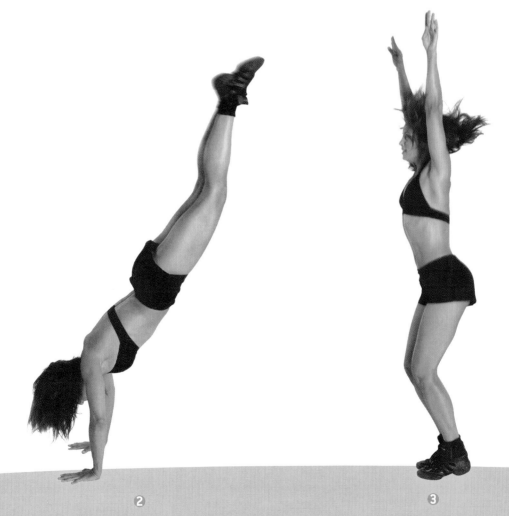

❷   ❸

Levels: 1–5

I love this exercise when I need to focus on the triceps. This is also a favorite when I'm trapped in a hotel room.

1. Stand in between two sturdy chairs that are facing each other. The chairs should be set far enough apart (about 3 feet [0.9 m]) so that you are able to move into the next position.

2. Your arms, straight down by your sides, should be on the seat of chair 1, and the heels of your feet on the seat of chair 2, with your legs straight and your body facing upward.

3. Slowly lower yourself down between the chairs. Do not allow yourself to bend forward at the waist; keep those hips up!

4. Straighten your arms and raise yourself back into starting position.

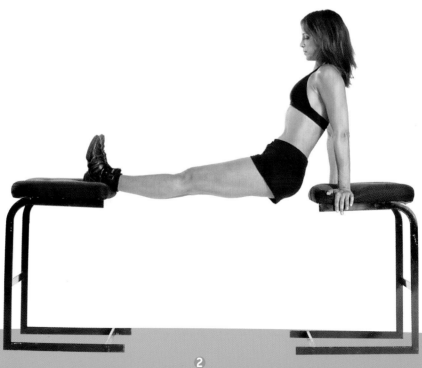

2

Variations:

- Keep your elbows tucked in close to your body to work your triceps more.

- Rotate your elbows out to work the chest.

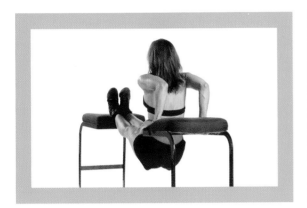

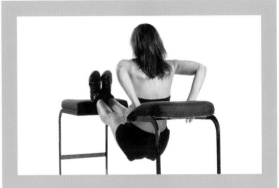

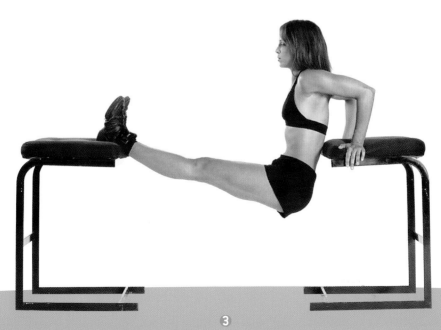

③

Abdominal Strengthening

Standard Issue Sit-ups

Levels: 1–5

Most people can do sit-ups, but frequently they do them incorrectly or mistake quantity for quality. Good form goes a long way toward good results.

❶ Lie on the floor, knees bent and legs hip-width apart. Securing your feet (under a couch or with a friend sitting on them) will allow you to make the most of this exercise. There are several options for arm placement, but the rule is never to use your arms to help you raise your torso. You should be focused on using only your ab muscles. I like to keep my arms by my sides.

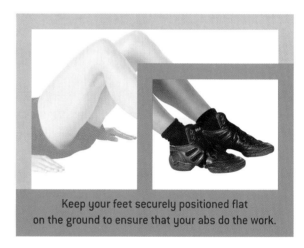

Keep your feet securely positioned flat on the ground to ensure that your abs do the work.

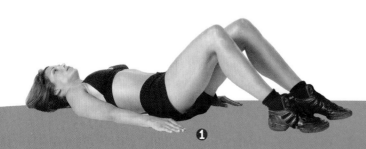

❶

2 Exhale as you bend at the waist to raise your torso up. Slowly come up, with your back flat and your chin lifting to the ceiling. Do not drop your chin! If your feet are secure, you can come all the way up until your chest nearly touches your knees.

3. When returning to your starting position, stay focused on your abs and slowly lower your torso.

Variation:
• To raise the difficulty level, place your left hand on your right shoulder blade and your right hand on your left shoulder blade so your arms are crossed behind your head.

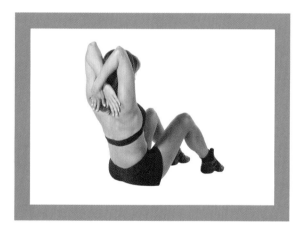

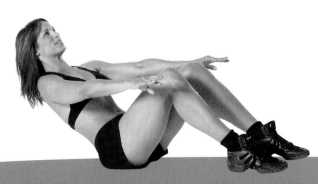

2

Abdominal Strengthening

The Twist

Levels: 1–5

Commonly known as bicycles, this exercise works more of the lower and side abdominals.

❶ Start by lying on your back, legs straight and fingers interlaced behind your head. During this exercise, never let your elbows come forward of your ears.

❷ Keeping your shoulder blades and feet off the ground, raise your left knee and twist your torso to the left until your right elbow meets your left knee. Do this exercise slowly, taking each motion as far as you can.

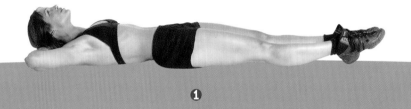

❶

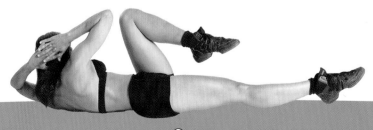

❷

❸ Now twist to the right, switching to your left elbow and right knee.

4. Using slow, deliberate movements, repeat steps 1 to 3 until failure.

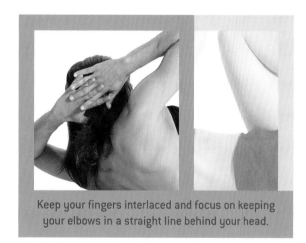

Keep your fingers interlaced and focus on keeping your elbows in a straight line behind your head.

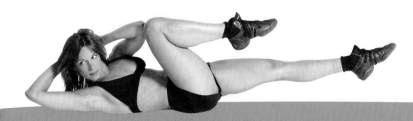

❸

Abdominal Strengthening

Windshield Wipers

Levels: 4–5

This exercise requires a stable horizontal support bar that can bear your body weight and allow you to hang from it. A chin-up bar would be ideal. With arms fully extended, your feet still should not touch the ground. (Oh yeah—these are really hard!)

1. Grab hold of the bar ("palms in" is the easier choice), and let your body dangle.

❷ Keeping your legs and back straight, bend at the waist to raise your legs as high as you can, keeping your legs together and tight the entire time. Your body will end up in a V shape.

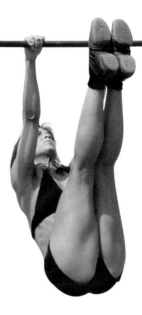

❷

❸ Keeping your legs up and your body still, shift your legs to the right as close to 90 degrees as possible.

❹ Now shift your legs to the left, again striving for a 90-degree angle.

5. Move slowly and repeat to failure. Don't stop 'til you drop!

Variation:
If steps 3 and 4 are too difficult, skip them altogether and stick to simply raising and lowering your legs as directed in steps 1 and 2. Go to failure!

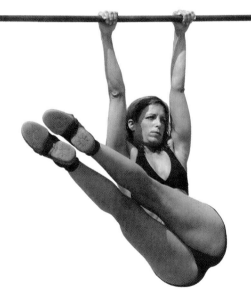

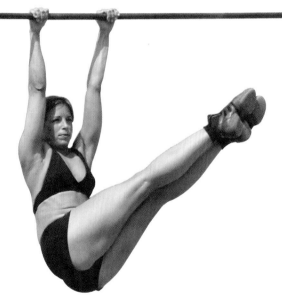

❸

❹

Abdominal Strengthening

Backflips

Levels: 4–5

I'm including this exercise because it's an excellent way to really work the abs, especially for people looking for something more exciting than what's at the neighborhood gym. Note that any of the gymnastics exercises in this book should be learned with an experienced spotter who will provide the support and guidance you need to take your body through the rotation. Backflips, in particular, are dangerous if you don't know what you're doing. Good form and technique are imperative.

❶ Start in a standing position, with arms slightly out and feet slightly apart.

❷ Swing your arms in front of you, reaching high to the ceiling as you explode off the ground. This reaching is important!

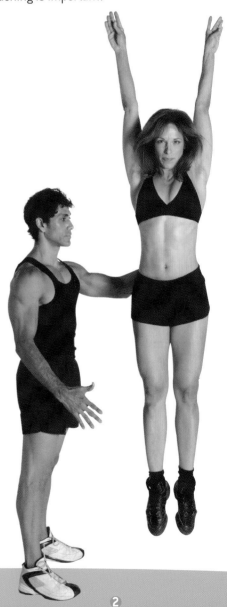

❶   ❷

Because this technique is called a backflip, a lot of people assume the motion is backward. You should think instead about getting as *high* as you can.

③ At the height of the trick, bring your knees up as tight as you can to your chest, wrapping your arms around your legs. The smaller the ball you can make of your body, the quicker your rotation will be and the more apt you are to make it around. Bringing your knees up is what causes the rotation.

④ Spot the ground, and open your body back up for a safe landing. This step is all about timing.

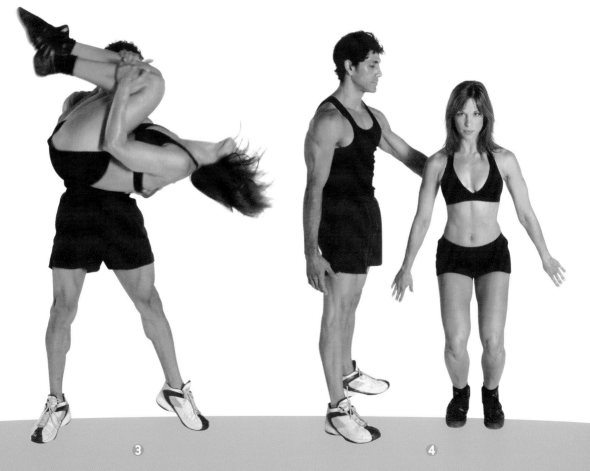

3

4

Chapter 2
Endurance

Endurance: *n.* the ability to last, continue, or remain; the ability to withstand pain, distress, fatigue, etc.; fortitude

By working on your endurance, you are working the most important muscle in your body: your heart. What could possibly be more important than that? Not only will a strong heart help you last longer in your Tae-bo class, it's also going to help you deal with the day-to-day stress that affects us all. To increase your stamina, you must focus on your cardiovascular system.

Our bodies are wonderfully fascinating. When you push your heart to work a little harder, your body produces endorphins. Now, these endorphins are magnificent little bits of happy magic. That's right; it's like your body is showering you with happy dust as a thank-you for being good to it. Your mood, your outlook, and your general sense of well-being are all positively affected by endorphin-producing exercise. Do you see how well your body responds to good deeds? If only you'll pay attention . . .

And that's not all, folks. In addition to feeling good and promoting a stronger heart, working your endurance is the quickest way that I know to lose weight.

For example, I wanted to lose a few pounds before starting the *Matrix* gig. After taking off a mere 7 pounds (3 kg), I noticed an incredible difference in my energy, especially when I went to do a tumbling pass or a fancy kick. All of a sudden, it seemed effortless. And then I thought about it this way: Imagine if I would have done that tumbling pass holding a 7-pound (3 kg) dumbbell. It suddenly made perfect sense. Five or 10 pounds (2.4–4.5 kg) may not seem like a lot of weight to lose, but if you think about carrying those dumbbells around with you everywhere, you'll begin to realize how much extra effort it takes to get through the day. And if you have 20 or 30 pounds (9–13.6 kg) to lose, imagine how much easier it would be to move through life if you could just get motivated enough to drop the weight.

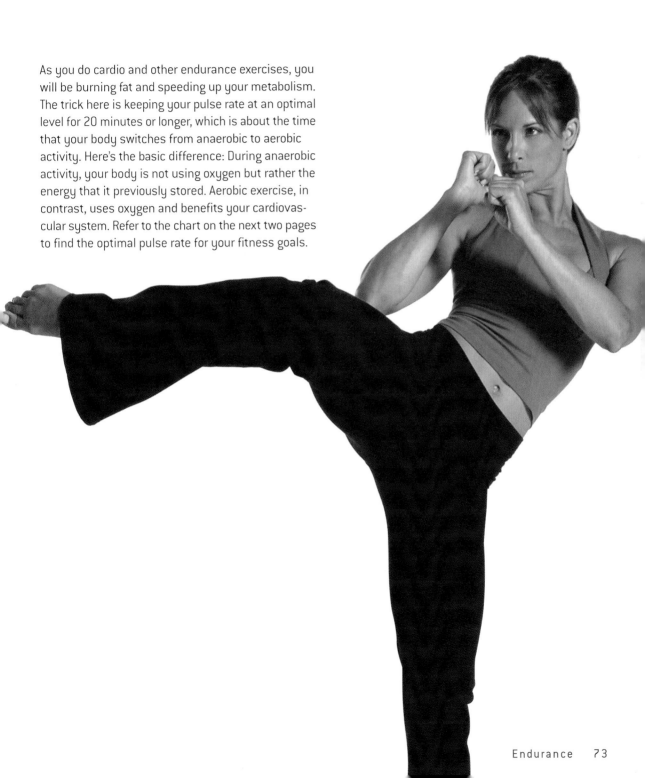

As you do cardio and other endurance exercises, you will be burning fat and speeding up your metabolism. The trick here is keeping your pulse rate at an optimal level for 20 minutes or longer, which is about the time that your body switches from anaerobic to aerobic activity. Here's the basic difference: During anaerobic activity, your body is not using oxygen but rather the energy that it previously stored. Aerobic exercise, in contrast, uses oxygen and benefits your cardiovascular system. Refer to the chart on the next two pages to find the optimal pulse rate for your fitness goals.

Target Heart Rate

These two charts provide a good guide to making the most of your workouts by working within your training "zone" (which depends on your age and level of fitness, from beginner to advanced). The chart below records the optimal heart rates (based on a percentage of your maximum heart rate) for your age group.

Age	Beginner 60%–70%*		Intermediate 70%–80%*		Advanced 80%–90%*	
	Beats/Min	Beats/10 sec	Beats/Min	Beats/10 sec	Beats/Min	Beats/10 sec
to 19	121–141	20–24	141–161	24–27	161–181	27–30
20–24	119–139	20–23	139–158	23–26	158–178	26–30
25–29	116–135	19–23	135–154	23–26	154–174	26–29
30–34	113–132	19–22	132–150	22–25	150–169	25–28
35–39	110–128	18–21	128–146	21–24	146–165	24–28
40–44	107–125	18–21	125–142	21–24	142–160	24–27
45–49	104–121	17–20	121–138	20–23	138–156	23–26
50–54	101–118	17–20	118–134	20–22	134–151	22–25
55–59	98–114	16–19	114–130	19–22	130–147	22–25
60–64	95–111	16–19	111–126	19–21	126–142	21–24
65–69	92–107	15–18	107–122	18–20	122–138	20–23
70–74	89–104	15–17	104–118	17–20	118–133	20–22
75–79	86–100	14–17	100–114	17–19	114–129	19–22
80–84	83–97	14–16	97–110	16–18	110–124	18–21
85+	81–95	14–16	95–108	16–18	108–122	18–20

*Percentage of maximum heart rate

Here you'll find the zone that corresponds to your fitness goal. When starting out, check your heart rate regularly to make sure you are working at an optimal level. Remember to continue to challenge yourself to make your efforts worthwhile.

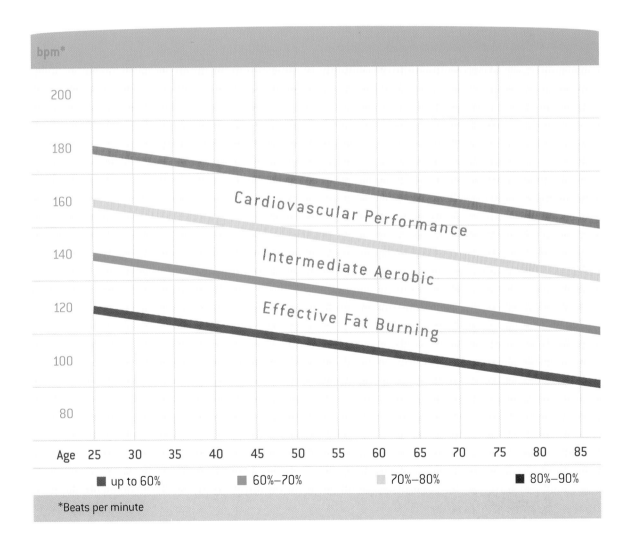

bpm*

■ up to 60%	■ 60%–70%	■ 70%–80%	■ 80%–90%

Cardiovascular Performance

Intermediate Aerobic

Effective Fat Burning

*Beats per minute

Exertion = Endurance

The heart is a muscle. We use a "resting pulse" to determine how in shape a person is (the lower the number of beats per minute, the more fit you are). The average resting pulse is around 80 beats per minute. Runners have a resting pulse in the low 40s. That means that non-runners are exerting double the amount of pressure and force to push their blood through the vascular system, whereas runners are so in shape that their hearts only need to pump 40 times to exert the same force.

Now, certainly in my crazy line of work, good stamina and a strong heart are the keys to success. Stunt-people put themselves in danger on a daily basis and must be able to cope with extreme stress. More than that, our actual physical endurance is put to the test time and time again. When you watch a huge fight scene, realize that sequence was performed many, many times in order to get it exactly right. Depending on the director, I have sometimes done more than 30 takes of one particular scene. And the thirtieth take has to be as high energy and strong as the first. It's not as if you can turn to the director and say, "Hey, I'm tired; think I'll go grab a power nap."

I did quite a few episodes of the WB's *Birds of Prey*, and for some reason, I always seemed to run into the same scenario. We would wait around the majority of the day, sometimes 10 to 12 hours, and then at the end of the shoot, at about 4 in the morning, when we were all tired and freezing, it would finally be time for the big fight scene. I loved the action on that show; it was always full of high-energy kicks and flips and taking out multiple bad guys. But in the middle of the night, let's face it: I'd rather be sacked out in my warm, cozy bed!

But just when I'd think I couldn't possibly do anything but curl up and go to sleep, I would be called in to do a big, dangerous stunt. Sometimes I'll be fighting five guys at a time, and the choreography is going at lightning speed. When we've done 10 or more takes, we are exhausted, and the chances of injury keep increasing. If anyone is so much as an inch off the mark, someone could get seriously hurt. That's why you'll often see the stuntpeople on set running in place, doing jumping jacks or whatever it takes to get the blood pumping and get ready to kick ass.

On film, we fight as fast and as hard as we can, because we want the director to like the take and move on. You have to give it everything you've got. In your life, too, you may often be in situations where you simply have to do things that you'd rather not do right then and there—exercise being one of them. But by keeping your body healthy and strong, you become capable of so much more.

It doesn't matter what level of cardio activity you start with. It's okay to start off slow. Just go for a walk every day and increase your distance and pace in small increments. Don't give yourself too big a task to accomplish. You'll be amazed at how quickly your body will respond. If you walk a mile (1.6 km), it won't be long before you're jogging a mile, and then running three miles (4.8 km).

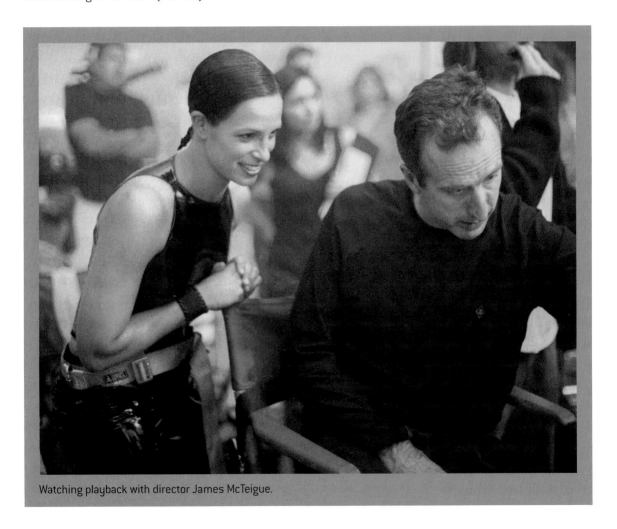

Watching playback with director James McTeigue.

Finding Your Cardio Bliss

If you hate running or are bored by those cardio machines at the gym, then find what suits you. I am a music lover, so dancing has always appealed to me. I also love my martial arts classes. They are both great forms of cardio. Then there are times when I have a lot on my mind, so I cherish a half an hour on a machine at the gym. It's the perfect time for me to process my thoughts or do a little problem-solving.

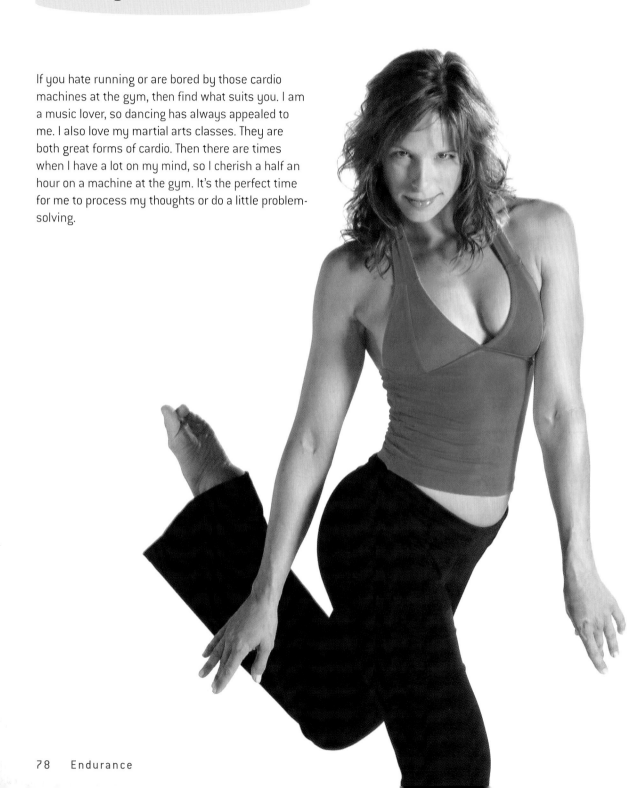

There's no rule that says you shouldn't enjoy being healthy. There are all kinds of activities that have already been organized and are just waiting for you to join in. There are bike tours that travel through national parks and wine country, hiking tours that are great social and sightseeing opportunities, and inline skating groups that help you discover your city in a whole new light. Opportunities abound to make cardio fun. If at first it seems like a chore, just give it a chance. Once you get into a new habit, I think you'll find that you'll quickly grow to love it.

Tip:
Commit early. Registering in advance for a race—runs, jogs, walks, bike races, triathlons—will provide additional motivation. The prepaid fee will give you a vested interest in following through.

Dance Fever

Dancing is a great exercise that not only builds up your cardio endurance but also is great for the spirit. I love dancing for its social aspects, too. You can go solo in a ballet, jazz, tap, hip hop, modern, or even belly dancing class, but if you've got someone to team up with, try some swing, mambo, salsa, waltz, or any other ballroom dance. Any of these dance forms will contribute to your coordination; some require more endurance, some more flexibility, and some simple strength. And just so you don't think that dancing is for pansies, remember that Bruce Lee himself was a champion cha cha dancer! Almost everyone has fantasized about learning one of these dance forms and unleashing a hidden talent. Which one appeals to you?

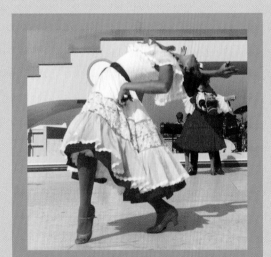

This is my first professional gig, as a World Dancer at Epcot Center in Orlando, Florida.

Exert Yourself

The human body is essentially the same as it was 5,000 years ago, but our society has switched from a nomadic, traveling state to a much more sedentary existence. Back in the day, our ancestors walked for miles, hunted, and did virtually everything by hand and on foot. These days, we drive cars, have our food delivered, and do virtually everything with the help of machines. Working out should be the norm for the human body, not just what fitness fanatics or extremely motivated people do. A sedentary environment is not normal and does not fit our physiology. If you're not doing anything physical, *that's* not normal. Our bodies are designed to move all day long. So let's find out how you can move yours!

If you use a/an:	Try this instead:
Elevator	Stairs
Escalator	Stairs
Moving walkway	Walk briskly
Grocery cart	Grocery basket
Wheelie suitcase	Carry your bags
Boardwalk to walk on	Walk on sand
Ramp	Stairs
Car to go less than 2 miles (3.2 km)	Walk
Car to go less than 10 miles (16.1 km)	Bike
Delivery service	Walk to nearby restaurant
Stationary bike while reading	Spinning class
Electric lawnmower	Push mower
Golf cart	Walk the course

Endurance Exercises

Cardiovascular workouts are the first and most important regimens you should do when you want to lose weight. If you're as much as 15 pounds (6.8 kg) overweight, do cardio exercise before you begin to build your muscle. The reason is simple: when you're overweight, you are putting excess strain on your body (joints, heart, lungs, systems). You want to lose the weight first so your body becomes more responsive. If you're severely overweight, make sure to consult a doctor, monitor yourself, and start out very slowly. Successive approximations are very important—meaning, take baby steps! If that means that you start off with a slow walk around the block, that's perfectly fine.

Exercise is a stressor, and if your body isn't in a good place, it can sometimes have a negative impact on your body. If you've only got 10 pounds (4.5 kg) to lose, it's not going to hurt you to do weight training in conjunction with cardio, but *only* lifting weights is not going to cut it if weight loss is a goal. Everybody is on his or her own path. The important thing is to work toward being healthier.

For each of the following exercises, there are two rules:
Rule 1: Warm up!
Rule 2: Pulse up!

Take a look at the chart on page 74 to see what your heart rate should be and then keep it up there for at least 20 minutes.

Food Philosophy

My view is simple: Calories in, calories out. In other words, food is fuel. The higher quality fuel we use, the better our performance. And for those times when we stray, vitamins and minerals make perfect plugs for the holes created by our poor dietary habits.

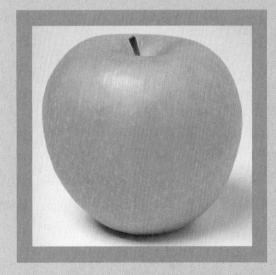

Endurance Exercises

Calisthenics Circuit

I'm often on set for up to 12 hours a day. When there's no time to work out, I try to find a corner or go outside and squeeze in a little endurance training. It's challenging to find activities that get my heart rate up and keep it up for at least 20 minutes. Doing a circuit of different activities can combat boredom. Here's a suggested "circuit":

Do each of the following activities for 1 minute each. Complete the full circuit at least four times. The goal is to get to 20 full minutes of activity.

❶ **Jogging in place:** If you're not needed at work for a half-hour, feel free to run wherever you want!

❷ **Push-ups** (see page 56): Shoot for 1 minute. If you are unable to do full plank push-ups, allow your knees to rest on the floor while still keeping a flat back.

Jogging in place

Push-ups

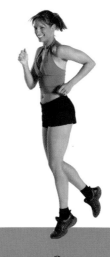

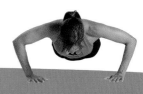

❶

❷

❸ Jumping jacks: Stay light on your feet and keep your body strong. Even this basic exercise should be done with good form.

❹ Shadowbox: Keep light on the balls of your feet, moving the whole time. Throw punches in the air in front of you, being careful not to fully extend your arm (which could strain your elbow). Mix it up with straight punches, jabs, hooks, upper-cuts—you don't have to have perfect form, but the idea is to keep your heart pumping.

❺ Knee jumps: Jump up, feet together, pulling your knees to your chest. Place your hands on your knees to help pull them toward your chest.

Variations:
Kicks (see pages 88–93): Rotate kicks into the circuit to liven up your workout.

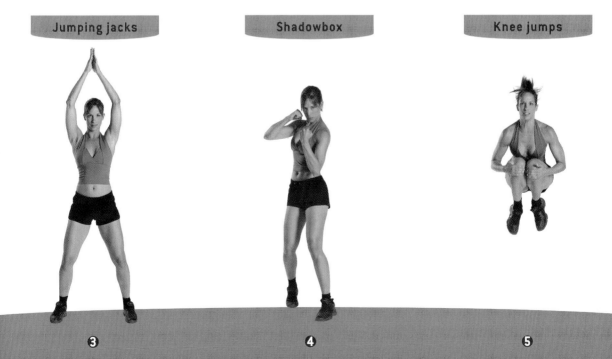

Jumping jacks · Shadowbox · Knee jumps

❸ ❹ ❺

Endurance Exercises

Get Your Groove On

Next time you're at the gym, take a look around you and see how many people on machines are reading magazines or watching TV and don't seem to be exerting any real energy. I would rather you spend half the time on a machine and be really focused on your workout. This exercise will give you a new approach even if you're on the same old machine.

1. Pick some music based on your mood. While something upbeat may seem preferable, any music that inspires you will work. A CD or iPod with a variety of tempos is going to be ideal.

2. Pick any cardio machine at the gym. It doesn't matter which exercise you choose—this is about letting the music drive you.

3. The key here is to lose yourself in the music. Let your feet keep up with the music. Keep the resistance as high as you can and still keep in time with the music. Basically, if the song is fast, you'll be working less resistance. If the next track is a little slower, increase the resistance.

I realize this sounds simple, but in order to maintain the challenge, follow this basic rule: Get the resistance up to where you literally can't keep up, then pull back one level at a time until it's doable. Make sure you check the heart rate chart on page 74 to ensure that you're performing optimally and safely.

Note:
Staying focused or losing yourself in the music for 20 to 30 minutes is a great stress releaser. Don't let thoughts about work or family stress get in the way. (See page 100 for focus exercises.) I think you'll find that you can withstand more time on a machine if you take your focus away from the work and channel it into something that inspires you—the way music does for me. And remember that the key to cardio is *duration of exercise*.

Endurance Exercises

Bleacher Blastoff

There are several ways to utilize a set of bleachers or a flight of stairs for an optimal cardio workout. Obviously, running up the stairs is a good way to start. From there, let's get creative:

- Double stride the stairs by hitting every other step.

- Try hopping up each step with legs together.

- Hop up each step one leg at a time.

- Hop up every other bleacher. (For this variation, be sure to pump with your arms for a little extra help.)

The key here is to mix it up to avoid boredom. If you're already a superstar athlete, carry some weights with you and see if that doesn't get your heart pumping.

Note: Running down a flight of stairs can be a bit dangerous, especially if you are tired. Give yourself a break on the way down: Take your time!

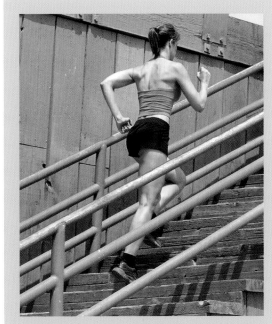

"Double striding" the stairs gives you an added cardio challenge.

H₂O

Water is one of the most important things I incorporated into my life after becoming a stuntwoman. The single best piece of advice I can offer to people looking to better their body is: Drink water, lots of it. I learned the following lesson from some Navy SEAL friends of mine who put me through a mini boot camp to train for an independent film I was working on. The saying may be crude to some, but still it remains an all-important motto: Piss clear. People in the military, top athletes, doctors, and anyone who prides him- or herself on being health- and body-conscious will tell you, your body is a tool and must be kept clean. Water not only hydrates you but also flushes out the impurities and toxins that build up, and it helps to keep everything functioning properly.

Many of us put all kinds of crazy things into our bodies. I happen to love coffee and realize that it's not exactly the healthiest thing for my body, so I allow myself my treat in the morning, and then I drink water for the rest of the day. Eight glasses a day is what nutritionists recommend.

In an average day alone, our bodies actually lose 2½ liters of water, all of which needs to be replenished. I keep water with me all day long and I just do the best I can. We are human: No one lives a perfectly healthful existence, and I certainly don't expect you to. But as much as you can, try to find a balance.

I hear so many complaints about people who hate the taste of water. I used that excuse myself. Any new habit takes a while to get used to. Be committed to making the change and know that after the initial few days, it will become pleasurable to you. Until then, add a wedge of lemon or lime and suck it up. Your body will thank you.

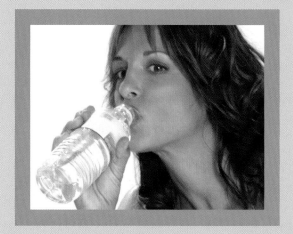

By keeping your body clean you are going to gain some bonus effects. You might see great changes in your skin, hair, and nails. Being so good to yourself will give you more energy and improve your overall mood.

Setting the record straight:

- Sorry, folks: Sparkling water does not count because of the carbonation. It doesn't flush the body in the same way as still water.

- Many hold a common misconception that salt makes you *retain* water. (Think about the irony of the stranded sailor dying of thirst in the middle of the ocean, knowing the salt water will dehydrate him.) After a strenuous workout, your body will tell you if it needs more water, sodium, or electrolytes. All you have to do is listen.

Running or jogging is probably the most common form of cardio exercise. *Fartlek training* (from the Swedish word for "speed play") is popular among serious runners: It involves alternating between long intervals of running or jogging and short intervals of sprinting. A good beginning technique is to alternate between two to three minutes of jogging and 30 seconds of sprinting. But if you're like me, this just sounds too boring. So let's add a little pizzazz to it.

1. Pick a destination (a neighbor's house, a coffee shop, your office, wherever). Get creative by making up different outdoor courses that will take you to your destination by routes around your town or neighborhood.

2. Sprint the straight areas and jog (or walk) the corners. This is a great way to get and keep your heart rate up while giving your muscles a break.

Tip:
Pick a partner and talk the talk while you walk the walk. Catch up on the day's news or gossip while you go running. If you pick a coffee shop as your final destination, you can treat yourselves for all your hard work.

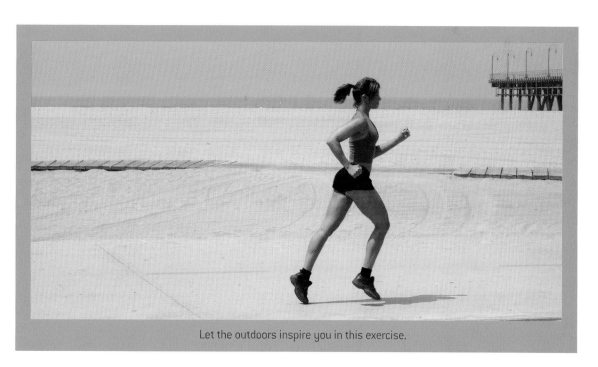
Let the outdoors inspire you in this exercise.

Follow the Leader

Partnering up with another person at a similar fitness level will help you keep to your workout schedule and will make you work harder. My partner and I do this exercise with martial arts kicks. However, if that doesn't work for you, you can make up virtually any high-energy movement to get the same results, including jumping jacks, cartwheels, sprints, or even silly dance moves.

1. Turn up some pumpin' music.

2. Stand face-to-face with your partner.

❸ Person 1 throws a kick.

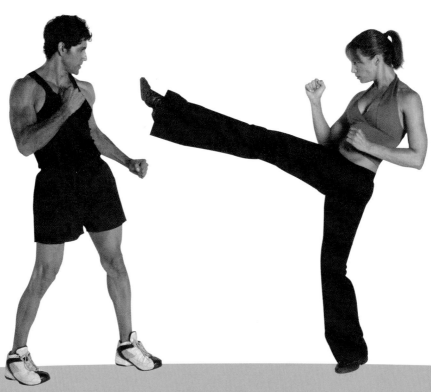

❸

4 Person 2 mimics that kick.

5. Person 1 throws a different kick, and Person 2 mimics again, and so on.

6. As you get going, alternate roles and create combinations of kicks for your partner to mimic.

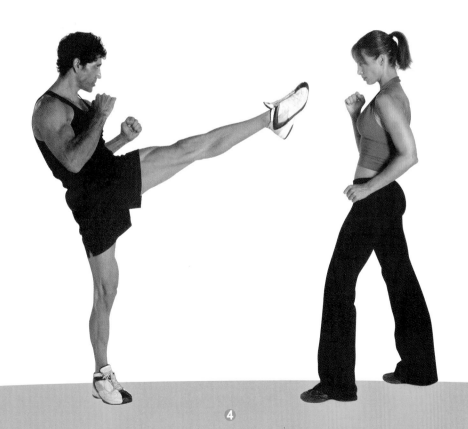

4

Kicks should come from a fighting stance: Start in a comfortable standing pose, feet hip-width apart, with your kicking foot slightly behind the other foot. Your knees should be slightly bent, as are your arms, and your hands should be in loose fists with your thumbs on the outside. If your right foot is back, your right fist should be to the right of your jaw and your left fist should be about a foot (0.3 m) in front of your left shoulder.

Now try these simple steps for some basic kicks.

❶ Start from fighting stance. Bring your right leg in front of you, bending at the knee. This position is called "the chamber."

❷ With a flexed foot, straighten your right leg in front of you, pushing out with the ball of your foot.

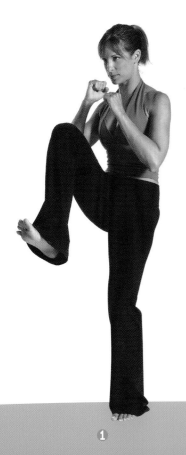

❶

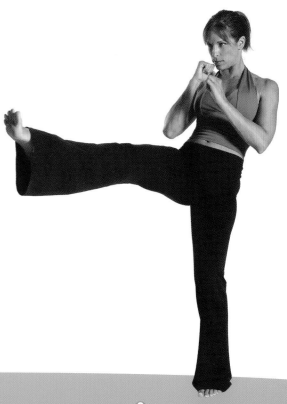

❷

❸ Return your leg to the chamber position.

❹ Return to your fighting stance.

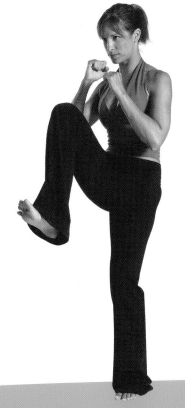

3

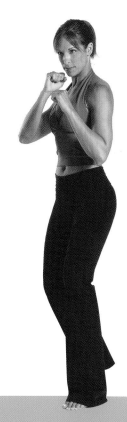

4

Roundhouse Kick

1 Start from fighting stance. Chamber your knee in front of you so that your hip is turned over and your knee is bent at a 90-degree angle. Your knee should be pointed to your left and your foot pointed toward the right.

2 Leaving your thigh where it is, unbend your knee so that your leg swings out in front of you as it straightens. Keep your foot pointed.

3. Rechamber your leg.

4. Return to fighting stance.

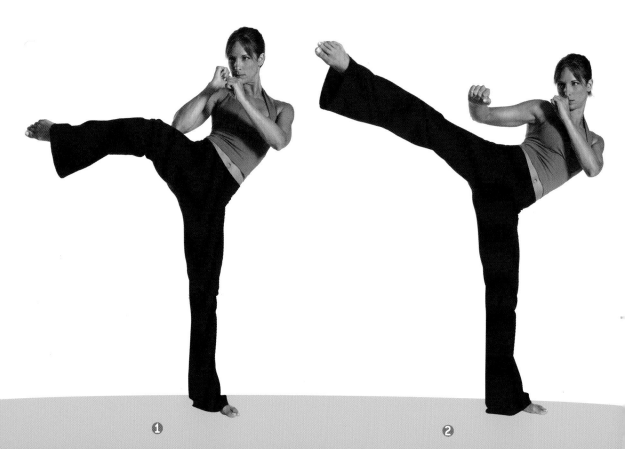

1

2

Endurance Exercises

Side Kick

1 Start from fighting stance. Bring your right knee up to your side with your hip turned over, your knee facing the front wall, and your flexed foot facing the right wall.

2 Extend your right leg by pushing out with your heel, keeping your foot parallel to the floor.

3. Rechamber your leg.

4. Return to fighting stance.

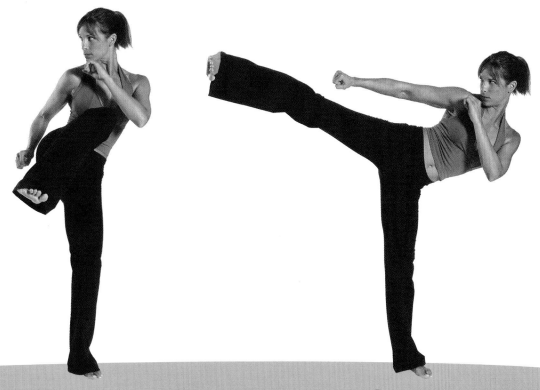

1

2

Chapter 3

Focus

Focus: *n.* concentrated effort or attention

Your overall agility is really what this book is about—that is, incorporating all of these skills to be at your overall best. But agility means more than just being able to maneuver efficiently. It also encompasses your ability to think on your feet, react in the moment, be aware of your surroundings, and adapt to the challenge at hand. And so it's important that we take on the topic of focus.

This book is mainly about getting physically fit through exercise. However, I believe that mind, body, and spirit are all interconnected, and it's of the utmost importance to have a clear head to accomplish what you want out of life. We work out to stay healthy and to deal with stress. And the psyche plays a huge part in achieving that goal.

People always think that stuntmen are grown-up versions of the little boy on your block who made a glider out of cardboard, plastic wrap, and glue and tied himself to the back of the UPS truck. Not true! The best stuntpeople are athletes who have good heads on their shoulders and can react quickly in the face of anything the situation demands.

So much of our job and our performance relies on trust—trusting one another *and* trusting our equipment. Oftentimes my safety is in the hands of my fellow stuntperson. And more often than that, my life depends on the equipment. Technology allows us to do increasingly outrageous things and remain safe. For example, when I was doubling Kate Beckinsale in *Pearl Harbor*, a decelerator (a machine that's used to simulate a freefall—it is designed to slow you down at the last second and keep you from splatting on the ground) was used to make it look like I was falling out of control when in reality I was perfectly safe. The key element is giving the trust over so that I can focus on the job at hand.

When a script calls for a dangerous stunt, chances are it's never been done before in exactly the same circumstances. And although we may be able to rehearse certain elements, we usually have to quickly assess the situation and then go for it when the cameras roll. It's important that we try to eliminate all removable hazards and then mentally prepare for all possible outcomes. We must also be acutely alert, because on a movie set you just never know what might happen.

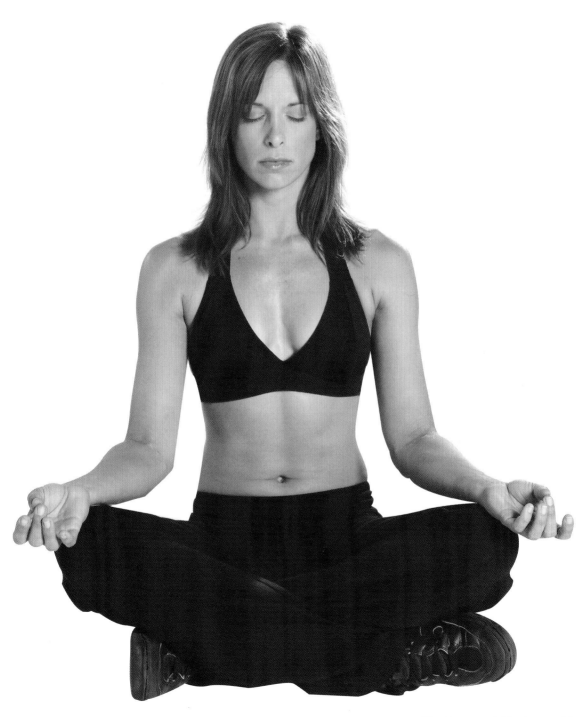

The Fear Factor

Let's address fear and adrenalin. Some people run in the face of fear, while others are adrenalin junkies. If there's an activity that you've always wanted to try but you've never been able to will yourself to conquer your fear, now's your chance!

Fear is an emotion that everyone experiences at one time or another, and it can manifest itself physically, often in the form of a panic attack. But most times fear can be overcome if you face it and prove to yourself that it's mainly a product of your mind. If you have a fear of heights, for example, I suggest you jump out of a plane (just don't forget the parachute). If your phobia is severe, however, successive approximation is the best approach. (In other words, baby steps.)

The best advice I have for overcoming fear is that you learn how to focus. Control your mind; don't let it control you. When you're in a threatening situation, find something else to focus on so that your brain doesn't have the chance to go into panic mode. Laughter really is the best medicine. If you're anxiety ridden, try poking some fun at yourself. As an added bonus, hysterical laughter works those abs!

The upside to fear is adrenalin. Your body will produce this hormone in situations of distress, danger, or risk. It provides an amazing rush that numbs pain and often offers additional strength you didn't know you had. It's what attracts so many people to extreme sports.

Once, when shooting an episode of *Worst-Case Scenario*, I encountered a little mishap that gave me a fascinating lesson in the benefits of adrenalin.

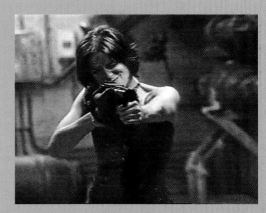

I got a burst of adrenalin from this web-shot gun, a powerful but non-violent weapon that shoots a net that wraps around its target.

We were shooting a sequence that involved my running on concrete in four-inch heels. (The glamour of Hollywood reminds me of my mother's famous words: "It's painful to be beautiful.") About 11 hours into the night, I could barely stand the pain in my feet. It was excruciating. During one of the takes, as I was chasing my bad guy down an L.A. street with what looked to be a grenade launcher, officers from the LAPD came screeching around the corner and drew their guns on me. It was terrifying being the mark of a loaded weapon. (I often have guns pointed at me, but never with real bullets.) As soon as the situation was under control—after being facedown on the cement—I stood up and became immediately aware that I had *no* pain. The crew was freaking out that I had almost been shot, but I was in awe over the fact that my feet didn't hurt—at all! About 15 minutes later, the pain slowly returned, but those 15 minutes of adrenalin were glorious.

Sometimes you can feel the effects of adrenalin for several hours. Six hours after being at the center of a huge explosion on the set of *Pearl Harbor*, I was still bouncing off the walls with a big grin on my face.

One of the most frequent questions I'm asked is, "Do you ever get scared?" The answer: "Hell, yes!" Here's a story for you. I landed my TV gig as Gear Girl on *Worst-Case Scenario*. This character was the show's co-host, whose role it was to demonstrate new and interesting gadgets. On my first day at work, I was asked to report to skydiving school. I had to do 25 jumps in only a few days to obtain my license so I could test an emergency parachute on the show. The day before filming, I finally did one rehearsal jump with the actual rig. Because of unforeseen circumstances, the chute opened so hard that it gave me third-grade whiplash and busted up my nose. It really scared me, and it really, really hurt.

After examining what caused the accident, I realized it was going to happen every time I pulled the ripcord. And so I thought of what I might be able to do in mid-freefall to lessen the blow. I basically found a way—through precision timing and body position—to brace my body mid-air to absorb some of the jolt. That could be the most serious concentration I've ever had to muster—not only to keep my mind on what needed to be done with incredible accuracy, but also to keep my mind focused away from my fear.

One of the things that I remember the most about that stunt was trying to get a grip on myself the night before. I was full of anxiety, and I knew I needed a really good night's sleep if I was to hit the stunt just right. And so on to our next topic . . .

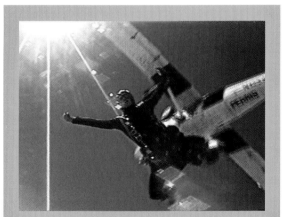

Gear Girl tests an emergency parachute—after only a few days of practice dives.

Sleep

The power of sleep extends far beyond helping you feel alert and awake. Our bodies literally require it for optimal performance in so many areas of our life, including learning, memory, and concentration. The average person sleeps seven hours a night, and a lot of people think that more than that constitutes laziness. But there's no shame in sleeping eight or nine hours! You may think five hours is enough for you, but you're kidding yourself.

Sleep is a key element to learning. Whether you're focusing on physical or mental skills, a solid night's sleep after learning something new is essential for retention. It's also been proven that sleep affects your cortisol level. Too much of this growth hormone can cause anxiety, depression, and fatigue. Proper levels help build lean body mass and burn fat. In other words, it has a huge effect on your mental and physical state. What else can make such a profound difference in your life—and require nothing more than your ability to let go and relax?

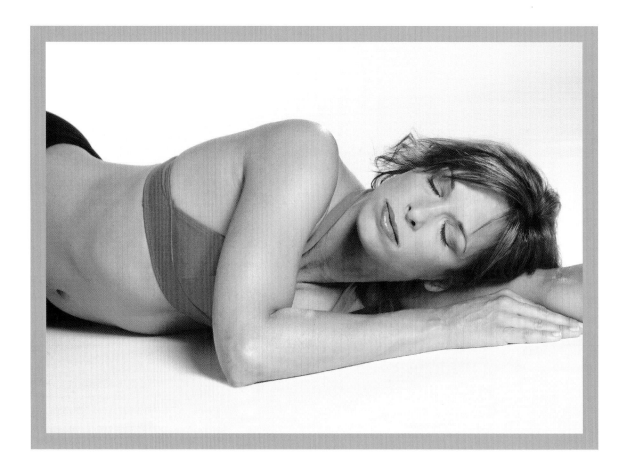

If I know I need a good night's sleep, I plan ahead. Exercising at the right time promotes sleep. Studies show that late afternoon is the prime time to exercise to ensure a good night's sleep. A hot bath is great for winding down before climbing into bed, as is anything that will help you relax. One great tip that I seem to hear over and over is that you should associate your bed with sleep and sex only. This isn't a place for paying bills! If you haven't fallen asleep within 20 minutes of going to bed, then get out of bed and try to relax until you are sleepy. Maybe you have too much on your mind. If so, jot down some of your thoughts to get them out of your head and onto the paper.

Some people think that if they need to go to bed early, they should stay up late the night before. I highly disagree. Don't ever willingly deprive yourself of sleep—you may get overtired and be less likely to sleep the following night. Here are some other basic but important sleep tips:

- Get your sleep whenever you can. If you can nap during the day, go for it. Twenty-minute power naps are awesome.

- If you know you have trouble sleeping, be extra wary of your daily caffeine and alcohol intake. Caffeine can stay in your system for up to 12 hours, so if you know you need to turn in early, cut out iced tea, soda, chocolate, and coffee after noon. Avoid alcohol; it's not a sleeping pill.

- Letting go of your logical mind will allow for greater clarity and efficiency of thinking. It might seem contradictory, but it's been proven to be true. The mind is the clearest just prior to and just after sleeping, because it's the time when we let go of our conscious mind and allow it to shift to the subconscious.

Focus Exercises

Just Breathe

Keeping a clear head helps me in all areas of my life.

The following exercises will help you focus your mind and relax your body, whether your goal is simple stress relief or you need to recharge your physical energy.

This simple technique can help you still your mind to attain mental clarity and help you get the sleep you need.

1. Sit in a chair with your arms and legs uncrossed, and your back straight. (You can also lie in bed on your back, with your arms at your sides and your legs straight or slightly bent.)

2. Close your eyes and focus on your breathing. Your breathing shouldn't be forced, held, or uncomfortable. As you breathe in through the nose and out through the mouth, your breath should *gradually* become deep and rhythmic.

3. Do not let your mind drift away from its focus on your breath. It sounds simple, but if you are doing this for the first time, it will be very difficult to focus on your breathing for more than a minute or two. You will get better with practice.

If you are doing this exercise to fall asleep, lie still and focus on your breathing until you fall asleep. If you're doing this for mental clarity, practicing this method as few as five minutes every day can improve your life tremendously.

Tip:
Try lightly placing your tongue behind your upper teeth. This technique is believed to create a better flow of energy through your body.

Focus Exercises

Let It Go

Even if I can still my mind, my body might not want to let go of the day's tension. So I use the following exercise to relax my body as well.

1. Begin as in "Just Breathe" on the opposite page. Sit in a chair or lie on your back.

2. Start out by focusing on your breath.

3. Now bring your focus to each body part, starting at your toes and moving slowly up to your head. Feel your feet getting heavy. Move slowly up your body, focusing on one area at a time.

4. Take your time when you get to your face. Relax the lips, jaw, eyes, and temples.

5. When everything is completely relaxed, you'll feel yourself sinking heavily into the chair or mattress. You'll even feel your body buzzing. When the tension is gone, return to focusing on your breath. Do not let your mind wander.

Tip:
If there is a particular muscle that won't relax, make it as tight as you can and then release it.

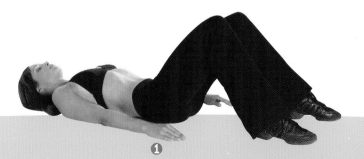

1

Tree Pose

One of the chief aims of yoga is to still the mind, and all of yoga practice benefits your ability to focus. Here are two poses for honing the mind-body connection and gaining mental clarity.

1. Stand strong and tall, with your big toes parallel to each other and your heels slightly apart.

2. Fix your eyes on a point directly in front of you and begin to concentrate on your breathing.

3. Shift all of your weight to your left foot, remembering to lengthen your spine toward the ceiling as you press your full left foot into the ground.

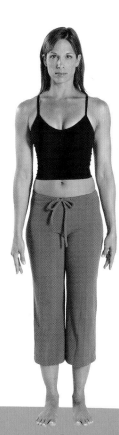

1

4. Place the bottom of your right foot to the inside of your left knee, maintaining your balance. If you are able, get your right foot as high as possible, pressing your heel into the left thigh.

5. Bring your hands together in prayer position in front of your chest.

6. Hold this pose as long as you can, maintain your gaze, and continue to focus on your breathing.

Variation:
If you'd like to challenge yourself further, continue the exercise by raising your hands above your head and allowing your focus to follow your hands.

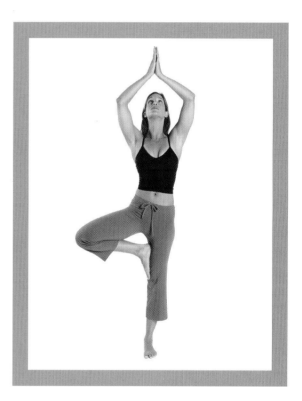

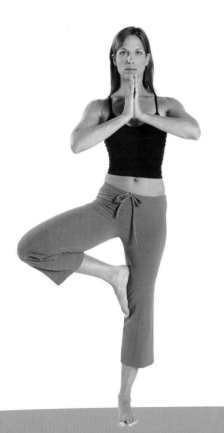

5

In addition to working your focus, this pose will give you a little extra stretch and strength for your legs.

1. Stand straight and strong, arms by your sides. Step your right foot about 4 feet (1.2 m) out to your side. Palms down, raise your arms so that they reach out to the sides and are parallel to the floor.

2. Turn your right foot 90 degrees to the right, making sure your thigh is turned out and the knee is over the ankle. Your left and right heels should be lined up. Keep your muscles tight and strong.

3. On an exhale, bend your right knee over the right ankle, so that the shin is perpendicular to the floor. Ideally, you want your right thigh to be parallel to the floor. You will find your balance by keeping your legs strong and pressing the outer left heel into the floor.

❹ Turn your head to the right and look out over your fingers.

5. Stay strong and straight in this pose, breathing deeply, for as long as you can. Rest, reverse feet, and repeat the pose.

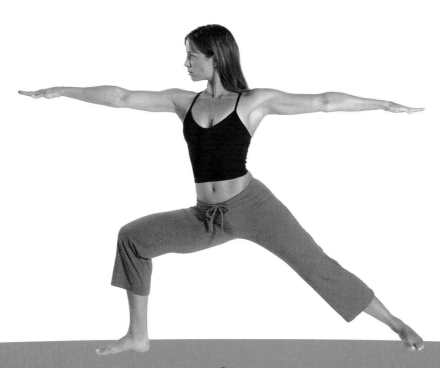

❹

Focus Exercises

Flame Focusing

Visualization is a great way to let go of stress and your daily thought process. A very simple way to start is to pick something that makes you happy—a sunrise, an ocean, a waterfall, a green field—and attempt to visualize it in your mind's eye. Generally, images in blues and greens work best because of their soothing qualities. Sometimes I prefer to focus on a tangible object first, so here's a basic visualization exercise to help bring your awareness to a state of relaxation.

1. Dim the lights and light a candle.

2. Relax and focus on the flame. Try to keep your mind from wandering.

3. After a couple of minutes, your mind should be quiet. At this point, close your eyes and visualize the flame in your mind.

4. Hold this vision for at least five minutes.

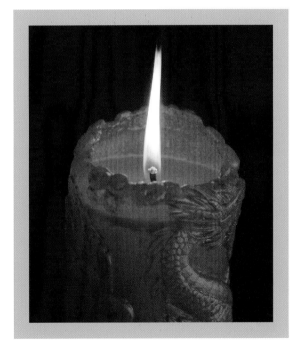

Focus Exercises

Mirror Image

Good athletes are able to move without thought, based on their sensitivity to the energy they receive from an opponent. Through this exercise, you will learn to sense and feel before your mind enters the equation. Do this exercise with a partner.

❶ Standing face-to-face with your partner, hold one hand up and have your partner mirror you, allowing your hands to touch. The lighter the touch, the more you are exercising your sensitivity.

2. As you move, your partner will follow you, maintaining contact with a light and steady touch. Keeping your arm movements fluid, start on a flat plane, but get dimensional over time by moving your hands forward and backward.

3. Close your eyes and continue to have your partner mirror your movements, this time simply by *feeling* the energy. Keep your touch as light as possible.

4. Now trade off and have your partner initiate the movement.

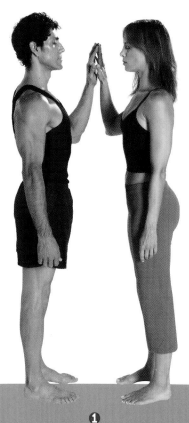

❶

Trapping

Here's a very basic exercise derived from the martial arts form known as wing chun (see page 109). These types of energy drills are fantastic. They're used by all types of athletes, including those you'd expect (boxers and fighters) as well as those you'd never expect to employ such techniques (including football linemen, who use this method to help them get through a line).

When doing this exercise, maintain your center-line energy. In other words, keep a straight and forward motion from the center of the body, and keep all movements inside the width of your shoulders.

❶ Both opponents start with the backs of their right hands touching. Your right leg should be forward and your right arm, held at shoulder height, should be bent in a wide V form.

❷ Your left hand pushes your opponent's right forearm down and forward. As you "trap" with your left hand, your right fist simultaneously punches straight toward your opponent's chest.

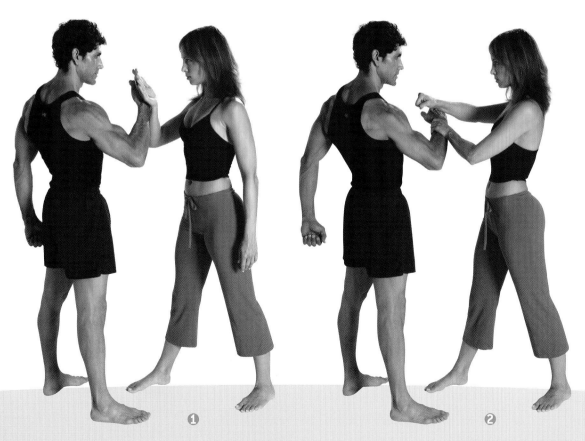

❶   ❷

❸ Your opponent's left hand parries the punch by pushing the back of your right wrist to the right and forward. Remember to stay within shoulder width.

❹ As you release your trap with your left hand, your opponent brings his wrist back to starting position, so that your right hands are back to back once again.

5. Repeat steps 1 through 4, this time switching roles.

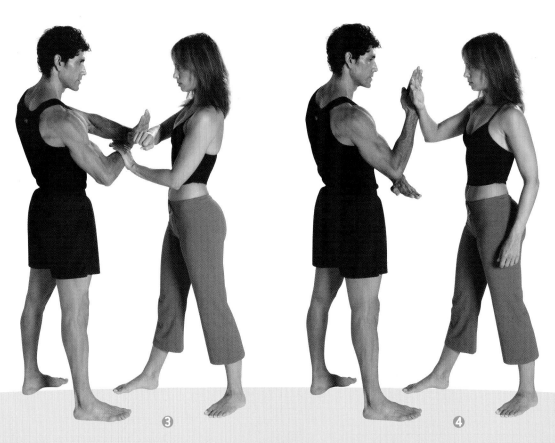

Start slowly until you find a rhythm. Ultimately, you should be able to close your eyes and begin to feel your opponent's energy. As you progress, work with different speeds.

Tip:
You can explore higher levels of this exercise by incorporating other blocks and punches with both hands. You will build confidence through repetition.

Sticky Hands

I want to turn you onto something called chi sao, or "sticky hands." This is a more advanced version of the mirror image exercise, but one of the most excellent sensitivity drills you can master. I wish I could share some of the technique with you, but it's simply too complicated to describe. You need to be taught and observed by an instructor. Chi sao derives from wing chun, a fascinating form of Chinese martial arts originally developed, according to legend, by a seventeenth-century Buddhist nun. It formed the core of Bruce Lee's martial arts foundation. Chi sao is all about fitting in with your opponent's energy and balance. I encourage you to check it out.

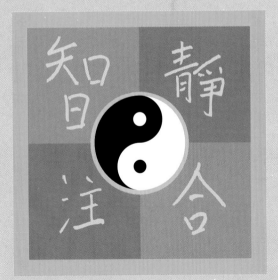

Chapter 4
Flexibility

Flexible: *adj.* 1 able to bend without breaking; pliant 2 adjustable to change; capable of modification

Flexibility is my strong suit. That's probably because I'm so passionate about it. We are usually good at the things we love to do. Even as a child, I was stretching constantly, always trying to get the perfect splits, and to this day, it is my favorite part of any workout. I can't imagine why anyone wouldn't want to take five to ten minutes a day to stretch, especially if they are feeling out of sorts, out of balance, or out of whack in any way. It's so easy, and it feels so good. I honestly believe that anyone who gives five minutes a day to stretching will see amazing results.

One of the things I love most about stretching is that it puts me in touch with my body. It's a great time for me to connect with myself, a time when I am inhabiting every part of my body. It's also a great way to relieve stress.

My approach is to focus on a particular muscle, breathe into it, and release it. I use my natural body weight to help me stretch and relax. You should never force or bounce into a stretch. What bouncing and forcing do, in fact, is make the muscle retract instead of release. Think of your muscle as a rubber band. Many of us have played with one, tugging and pulling only to release it and have it snap back. However, if you hold the band in a stretched position, you will see that it lengthens a little bit at a time, which is exactly what you want to do with your muscles.

Just get the muscle to its point of resistance, breathe into it, and then on your exhale, let your body weight sink into it more. Hold the position for a minimum of one minute, continuing to sink deeper into the stretch on every exhale. The longer you hold the stretch, the better your results will be. This technique, which we will discuss in greater detail later, is going to be very important in the exercises in this chapter.

My technique of stretching and controlled breathing comes from years of study as a dancer with various teachers from all over the world and from yoga classes that I have come to adore. I am by no means a yoga instructor, but I am someone who has experienced the benefits of this practice firsthand. If yoga is something you've been curious about, I highly recommend you give it a try.

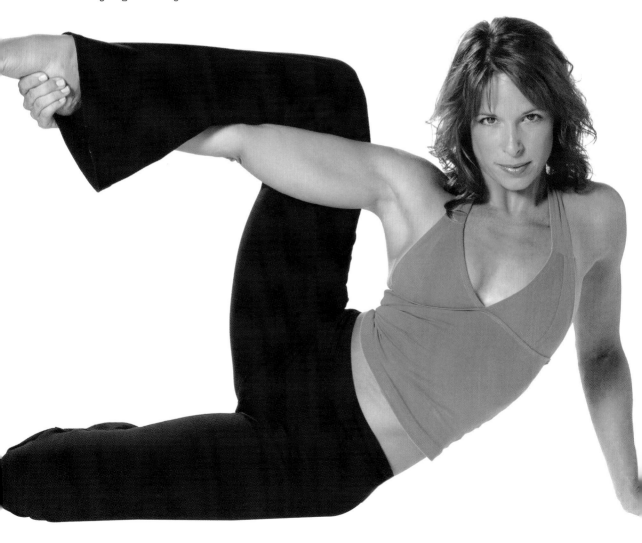

My Stretching Specialty

My flexibility is one of the main factors that have contributed to my success in the stunt business. Most stuntpeople have a specialty, and I have become known for my fight skills.

Being flexible helps me make things look, well, *flashy*. I can easily kick the face of the big bad guy who's 6′3″ when I'm only 5′7″. That was a big factor in making it through the *Matrix* audition, a very private, invitation-only event. We had to fight, we had to flip, and we had to "take reactions"—that is, when someone threw a punch, I needed to show convincingly how a body would react to it. For example, if Agent Smith were to throw an uppercut, how would my body go flying through the air? I can't just hurl my body in the air and splat it on the ground. There is a very specific technique to taking the blow without hurting myself. My flexibility and coordination are what allow me to get up off the floor and do it again and again.

While writing this book, I was called to do an episode of *Crossing Jordan*, and this technique came into play. They needed a stair fall. Generally, these suck, because no matter what, I'm sure to get bashed up. But because I'm highly flexible, I can contort my body into crazy positions without seriously hurting myself. In this particular case, it was important for me to hit certain points of an 18-foot (5.5 m) staircase, due to the crime scene evidence written into the script. I got tossed down five times and walked away unscathed.

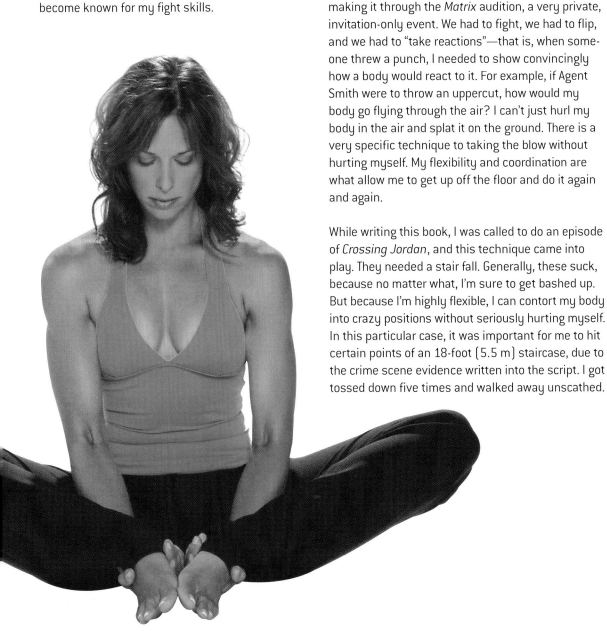

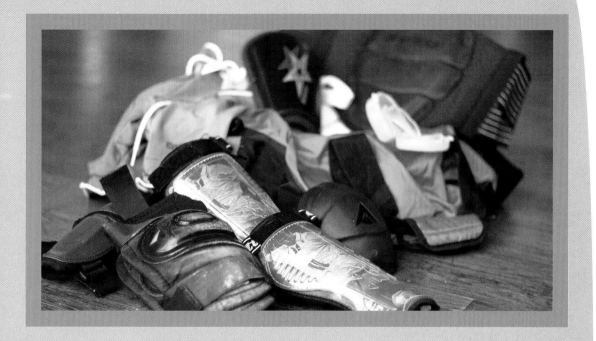

What's in the Stunt Bag?

I always tote a duffle or backpack to sets. The bigger the stunt, the bigger the bag. It's loaded with all kinds of equipment and protective gear:

- Protective pads that cover specific body parts (knee pads, elbow pads, back pads, shin guards, tailbone pad, and hockey girdle)

- Neoprene or thin foam to cut out customized padding (for a little extra protection when the wardrobe is too tight or too skimpy for regular pads)

- Mouthpiece (protects against broken teeth during car hits or car crashes)

- Ankle and knee braces (to provide extra support to those all-important joints)

- Medical tape (for securing Neoprene or for taping weak ankles)

- Straps and bungee cords (good extras that come in handy when you have to do creative rigging)

- Harness for wire stunts (worn under the wardrobe, it's what the wire clips onto)

- Flashlight (for dark sets and night shoots)

- Toy cars and action figures (to choreograph car chases or stunts)

- Black tennis shoes (for when I can convince a director to let me wear them in lieu of high-heeled shoes)

- And last but not least, I always bring my own medical kit (see "The Stuntwoman's Medicine Cabinet" on page 21)

The Stuntwoman's Rolodex

Here are a few category entries from my Rolodex. Sometimes I need to look outside to get help from specialists, and there are a number of people and places I rely on to help keep me in top form.

- **Acupuncturist**
  Acupuncture, which uses tiny needles to stimulate certain points on the body, has been around for thousands of years and has been used to treat everything from pain to chronic injury.

- **Chiropractor**
  Your bones need to be in their proper places for optimal healing. If you know you've tweaked yourself out of alignment, visit your chiropractor. He or she will use hands-on manipulation techniques that focus on the structural parts of your body (particularly the spine) to encourage overall health of the joints, bones, and connective tissue.

- **Dance studio**
  My favorite place to incorporate work and play. A high-energy dance class is a great overall workout that encourages strength, endurance, flexibility, and coordination. (And it's fun!)

- **Massage therapist**
  I prefer deep-tissue or sports therapy massage, which breaks down scar tissue, but you can also try Swedish or Shiatsu for general relaxation.

- **Reiki**
  An alternative therapy technique used to channel healing energy into your body.

- **Spas**
  The perfect way to treat yourself. I don't know about you, but I love treats!

- **Sporting goods store**
  The place to buy athletic shoes, hand weights, chin-up bars, athletic equipment, clothing, or gear specific to your sport.

- **Yoga center**
  Best place for integrating mind, body, and spirit.

- **Various friends**
  I'm constantly putting calls out to my friends to go hiking or skydiving, play tennis, or whatever. Any activity is more fun when you have a buddy along to share it.

One of the biggest workout mistakes I see is people getting too focused on building muscle and forgetting the importance of stretching. Building the muscle is great, but you must take the time to stretch it out. Smart body builders train using full range of motion (which means they fully extend their muscles during every strengthening exercise). The more you stretch a muscle, the fuller the muscle belly can get. As you produce muscle mass, you tighten that area of your body. It's important to stretch so that you don't lose full motion in your joints.

People trip and fall all the time. In life, accidents happen. But the more flexible you are, the less likely you are to get hurt. And in anything athletic you do, you'll be that much better at it if you are limber.

Whether you have five minutes or an hour to devote to your flexibility, do it. You will see results in no time. It will bring awareness to your body, and it's great for releasing tension and muscle knots. It's going to help with your overall agility and your ability to move through life. And it's incredibly self-rewarding.

Once you get in tune with your body, you will be able to tell which muscles always get tight. When you get the hang of the basics, you will eventually be free to improvise and create your own stretching routine. This will come in handy when, for example, you encounter one of those muscles you never knew you had. Slowly move around to find the position that will hone in on that muscle, and then use your own body weight to deepen into a stretch.

There are some good basic stretches in "First Things First" (see pages 22–33). Here, we are going to spend a little more time and effort to increase our flexibility.

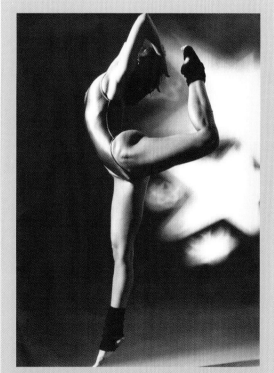

My stretching ability has allowed me to perfect my form, whether in dance or on the set.

Shoulder Flexibility

Stretch 1

Our poor shoulders are so often neglected. Shoulder exercises are of the utmost importance, especially if you are participating in any sport that involves throwing. Continuous abuse without stretching can result in a decreased range of motion.

All of these stretches start at a beginner level, and some of them progress to a more advanced level. Listen to your body. I want you to challenge—not injure—yourself. Decide for yourself if you're ready to take the next step.

❶ Grab hold of the end of a towel with your right hand.

❷ Place your right hand at the nape of your neck.

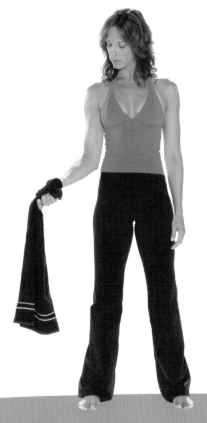

❶

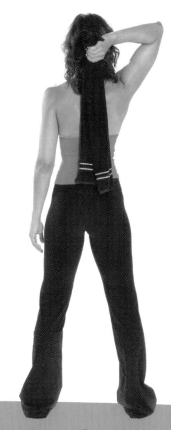

❷

❸ Place the back of your left hand against your lower back and grab the other end of the towel.

❹ With your right hand, gently pull straight up. Do not allow your left shoulder to roll forward.

5. Hold this position as you take several slow, deep breaths. Focus on releasing the tension on each exhale.

6. Reverse your hand positions this time, repeating steps 1 through 5.

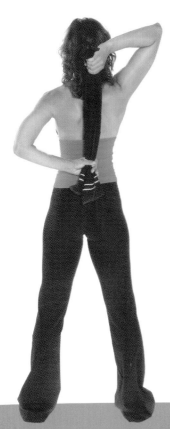

❸

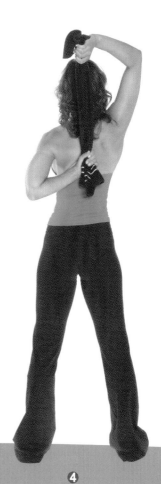

❹

Shoulder Flexibility

Stretch 2

1. Raise your right arm straight up above your head.

2. Bend at the elbow so your right wrist is behind your head.

3. With your left hand, gently pull your right elbow toward your left side.

4. Hold this pose and breathe.

5. Repeat steps 1 through 4, this time beginning with your left arm.

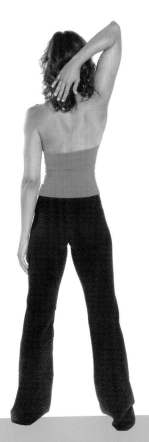

2

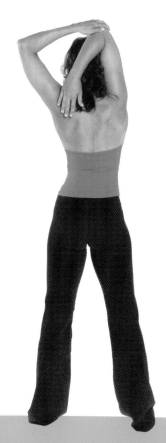

3

Shoulder Flexibility

Advanced Stretch

If you are already flexible in your shoulders, you should be able to combine the previous two exercises.

1. Raise your right arm straight up above your head.

2. Bend at the elbow so your right wrist is behind your head.

3. As in Stretch 1, reach your left arm behind you, but this time place the back of your left hand against your *upper* back.

4. Interlock your fingers.

5. Hold the pose for several long, deep breaths.

6. Repeat steps 1 through 5, this time beginning with your left arm.

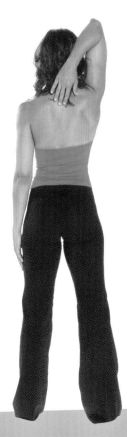

2

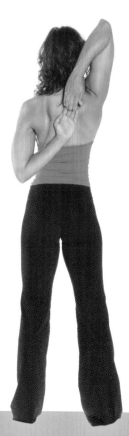

4

If you suffer from hip pain, it's quite possible that I'm about to make you very happy! These are simple, feel-good stretches that will open up those hips. For me, there is nothing more important than maintaining mobility in my hips, as my martial arts skills, especially, depend on it.

❶ Sit on the floor with your feet straight out in front of you. Be sure to sit straight and tall. Your hands can be on the floor by your sides.

❷ Bend your right knee and place the bottom of your right foot on the inside of your left knee.

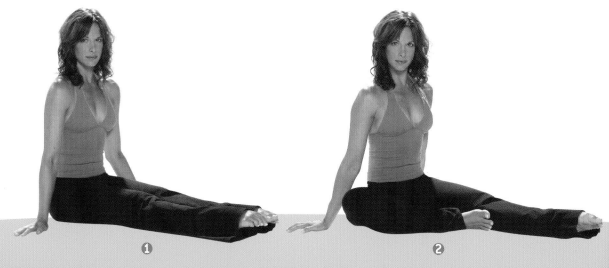

❶　　　　　　　　　　　　❷

3 If this is too easy, try placing your right ankle just above your left knee.

4. Take several deep breaths, releasing more of the right hip's tension on every exhale, gently allowing the right knee to sink closer to the floor.

5. Repeat steps 1 through 4, this time beginning with your left knee.

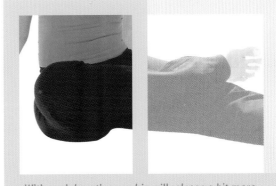

With each breath, your hip will release a bit more, and your bent knee should sink to the floor.

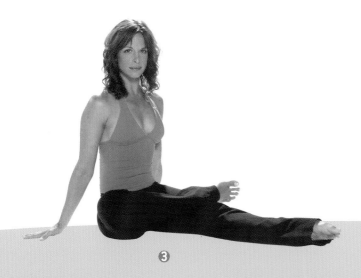

3

The last exercise may have been challenging enough for you. It really depends on the individual. You and only you will know how far to take things without hurting yourself. Stay focused, and be sure not to force these muscles. And if you want a little more stretch, here you go.

❶ Sitting straight and tall, bend both knees so that they point outward and the bottoms of your feet are touching.

❷ Place your arms in between your legs and under your feet, holding onto both ankles and bringing your feet as close to your body as possible.

3. Hold this position for a few inhalations and exhalations.

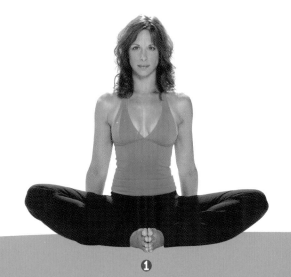

❶

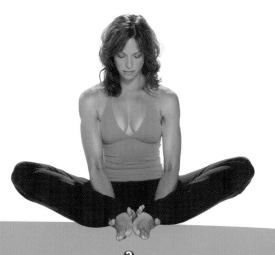

❷

4. Now place your hands in front of you and begin to walk them forward, allowing yourself to bend at the waist.

❺ Walk your fingers as far forward as you can, ideally placing your elbows on the floor.

6. Take a deep inhalation, and on your exhale, try to inch your fingers a little farther forward.

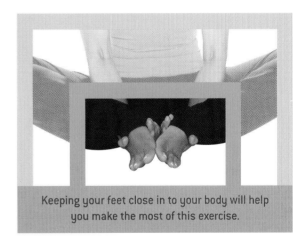

Keeping your feet close in to your body will help you make the most of this exercise.

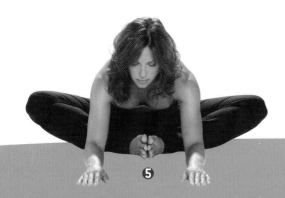

❺

Some people naturally have very open hips, and it can be tough to find a stretch that will work this area sufficiently. So if those last stretches weren't enough for you, Gumby, try this more challenging one.

❶ Sit with your legs in a triangle: your right foot positioned directly on top of your left knee, and your left foot directly beneath your right knee.

2. Hold this position for a few seconds and breathe.

❸ Now walk your hands out in front of you, allowing yourself to bend at the waist, and place your elbows on the floor.

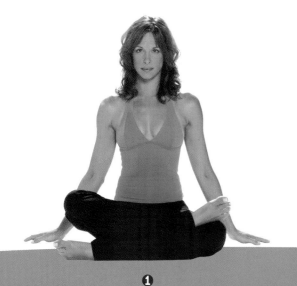

❶

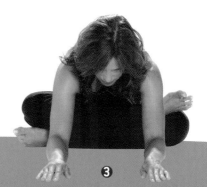

❸

4. Breathe, breathe, breathe.

❺ Switch legs so the left foot is now on top of the right knee, and repeat steps 2 to 4.

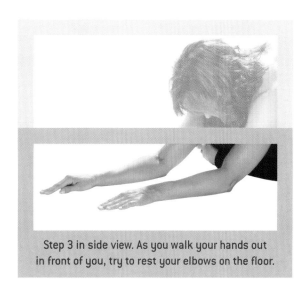

Step 3 in side view. As you walk your hands out in front of you, try to rest your elbows on the floor.

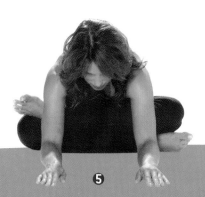

Thigh Flexibility

Stretch 1

If you've done the warm-up on pages 32–33, you've already started to increase your quad flexibility. If that is not enough stretch for you, here is an advanced version.

➊ Sit on the floor with a straight back and both legs straight out in front of you.

➋ Grab your right ankle, bend your knee, and put your foot as close to your right hip as possible. You will be sitting on your right shin. Place your hands on the floor by your sides.

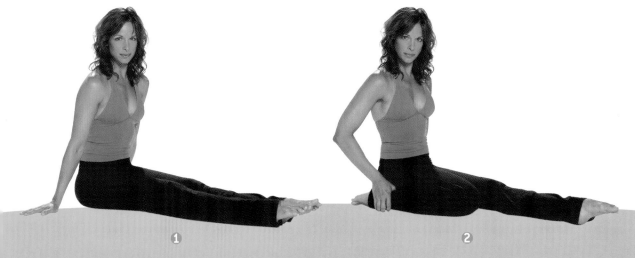

➊   ➋

3 Lean back, placing your elbows on the floor. Make sure you keep your right knee on the floor. If you are very flexible, you should be able to lie flat on your back. If so, be sure to keep your back from arching.

4. For a deeper stretch, keep both knees squeezed together.

5. Hold this position for one minute.

6. Now repeat steps 2 to 5, this time beginning with your left ankle.

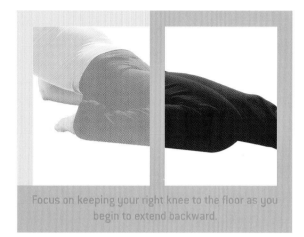

Focus on keeping your right knee to the floor as you begin to extend backward.

Variation:

If you feel comfortable taking this exercise to the next level, try folding both legs under at the same time, with your back on the floor. Remember to keep the knees together and on the floor.

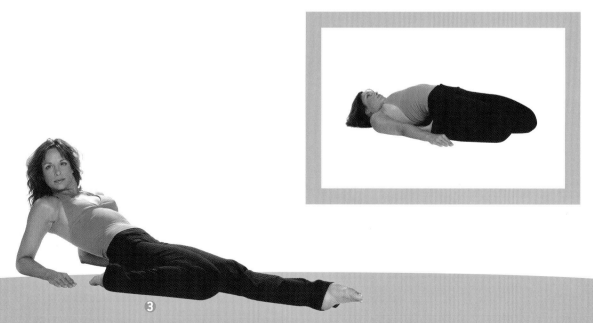

Your glutes (aka your butt muscles) take a lot of abuse, and people often neglect them. They are especially important to focus on if you are looking to increase flexibility in your lower back (they are connected, after all).

1. Sit on the floor with your right leg bent at a right angle in front of you. Your ankle and knee should rest on the floor. Tuck your left leg behind you.

❷ Hold your right foot with your left arm to keep it from sliding in. Your right arm can be by your side for balance.

3. Keep your body squared to the front and make sure you maintain a right angle with your right leg.

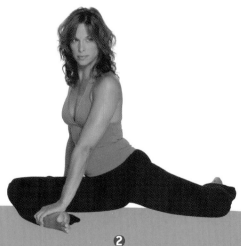

④ Slowly lean forward to increase the stretch.

5. Repeat steps 1 through 4, this time beginning with your left leg bent in front of you.

Variation:
Once you've mastered this exercise, take it a step further by straightening your back leg. Make sure to keep your hips squared to the ground. To make this position more comfortable, try placing a pillow under your right hip for support.

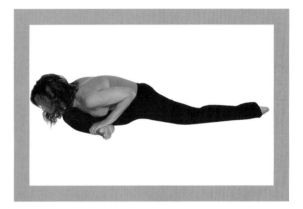

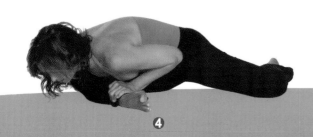

I hear so many people complaining about back pain. A little effort toward stretching will go a long way toward alleviating your suffering, especially for those of you who sit or stand all day. Give your back a break and try these exercises.

❶ Lie on your back with your feet on the floor and your knees bent and together.

❷ With arms out to your sides, turn your head to the right and drop your knees to the left.

3. Keep your right shoulder on the floor and breathe.

4. Repeat steps 1 to 3, this time turning your head to the left and dropping your knees to the right.

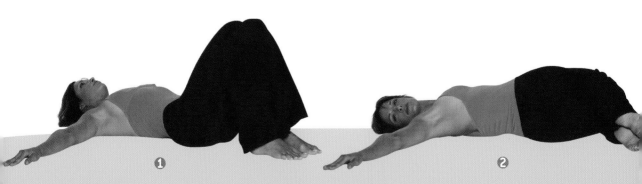

❶   ❷

Back Flexibility

Stretch 2

Now let's go deeper.

1. Lie on your back, knees bent, feet flat on the floor. Your feet should be slightly more than hip-width apart for balance.

❷ Bend your arms so your palms are flat to the floor next to your ears. Your fingers should point down toward your toes.

❸ Press up, pushing your stomach to the ceiling and keeping the weight equally distributed between your hands and feet.

4. Hold this pose for a few seconds and then slowly lower your body back down.

5. Repeat this movement several times. Each time you press up you should try to rise higher and stay up longer. You should feel the stretch not only in your back but on the entire front of your torso.

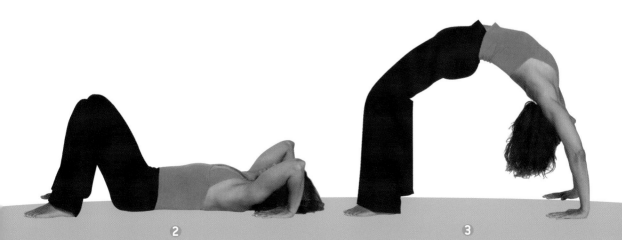

2

3

Mucho more stretch . . .

1 Repeat the preceding exercise (steps 1 through 3) with knees and feet together.

2 Once in the bridge position, lower your elbows to the floor, gently placing the top of your head on the ground.

3. Hold for several seconds, making sure to keep your pelvis pressed upward.

4. Slowly lower your body back to your starting position and repeat.

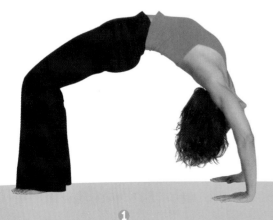

1

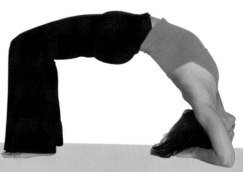

2

Hamstring Flexibility

Stretch 1

❶ Sit on the floor with your legs straight out in front of you.

❷ Take a deep inhale and reach your arms above your head, lengthening your spine away from the floor.

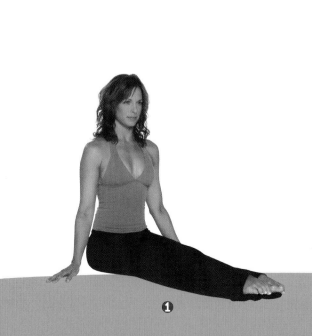

❶

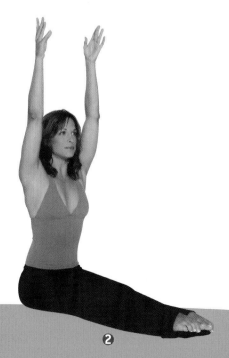

❷

3. As you exhale, slowly bend at the waist, keeping a flat back as long as possible, then fold your torso over your legs. Your hands should cup the outsides of your heels. Keep your belly button as close to your thighs as you can.

❹ Give a slight bend to your right knee on the inhale, then straighten and hold on the exhale.

5. Give a slight bend to your left knee on the inhale, then straighten and hold on the exhale.

❻ Stay folded over at the waist, with two straight legs, and sink deeper on every exhale.

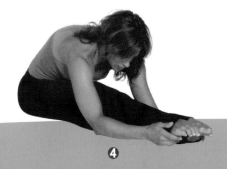

❹

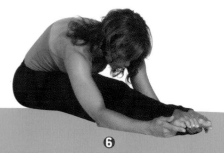

❻

Hamstring Flexibility

Stretch 2

So you say you want more?

1 Following steps 1 to 3 in the preceding exercise, come back to an upright position with your back flat. Inhale, then flex your feet so that your heels come off the floor. Your hands can be by your sides, or for a deeper stretch, grab hold of your toes and pull them toward you.

2 As you exhale, point your feet and round your back, gently pulling your chest toward your thighs.

3. Continue deep breathing and repeat.

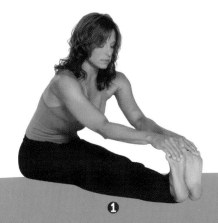

1

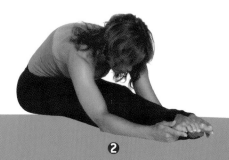

2

Inner Thigh Flexibility

Stretch 1

1. Sit on the floor with your legs in a wide V in front of you.

2. Place your hands behind your hips.

❸ As you inhale, lift your butt off the floor and move your hips forward, widening your V.

4. As you exhale, lower yourself back to the floor, making sure your knees are facing the ceiling. Do not let them roll in!

5. Take a few breaths, releasing the tension.

6. Repeat steps 3 to 5.

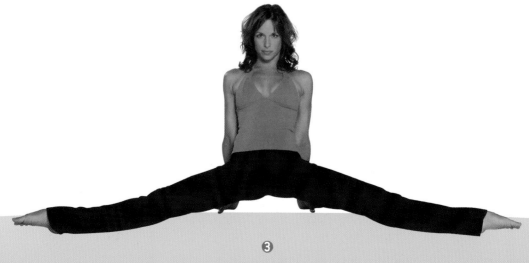

❸

7 To go deeper, place your elbows on the floor in front of you. Don't forget about those knees: They should not roll inward at any time.

Variation:
You can get more out of this stretch by facing a wall. When your legs reach 180 degrees, congratulations! You have graduated to a Chinese Split!

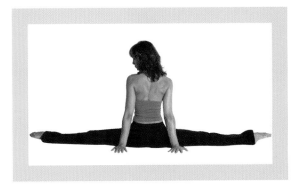

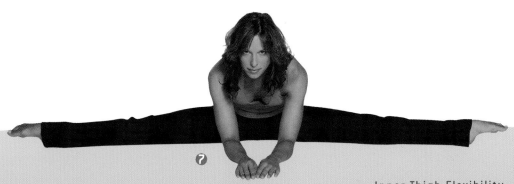

The Splits

Now that you're feeling all limber, you might want to go off and join the cheerleading squad. If so, you'll need to master these stretches!

❶ Sit on the floor with your right leg in front of you, your left leg behind you, and your weight on your right arm.

❷ Slowly straighten both legs outward in opposition.

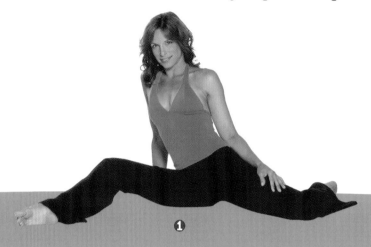

❶

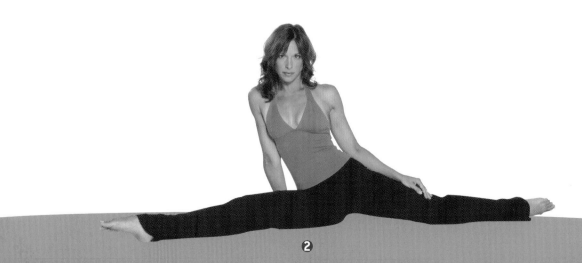

❷

❸ Keeping your torso forward, shift your weight to the center, placing both hands to the floor for balance. Remember to stretch to the point of resistance, then breathe deep and let your body's weight do the work. *Do not force, do not bounce*! When you reach this ultimate stretch, your hips should be squared to the front, your right knee should face the ceiling, and your left knee should be facing the floor, with weight on the quad.

4. Reverse legs and repeat steps 1 to 3.

Tip:
While training for the splits, never rise up. I don't want you to put weight or pressure on your back knee. Simply roll as far toward the center as possible while keeping your hips on the floor. You will eventually be able to roll all the way to the center.

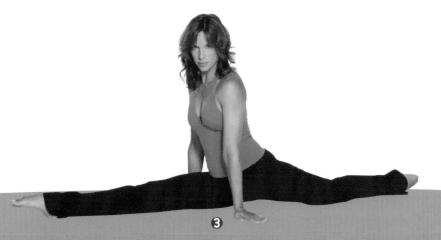

❸

The Splits

Stretch 2

One more impressive stretch will help you look like the limber superstar that you have become.

1 You will begin in a full split position, with your arms at your sides and hands on the floor for support.

2 Once in your full split, bend the back leg, cupping your foot to raise it toward the ceiling.

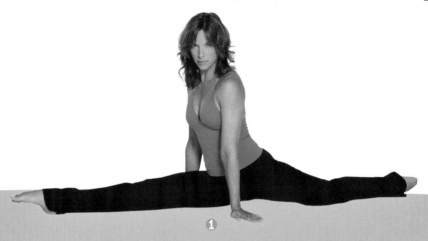

①

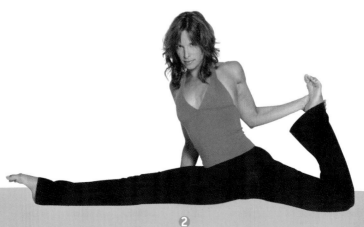

②

3. Continue to pull your foot toward your lower back.

④ Reverse legs and repeat.

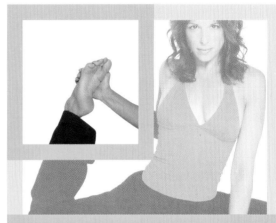

Firmly cup your back foot and on each exhale exert slightly more pressure to increase your stretch.

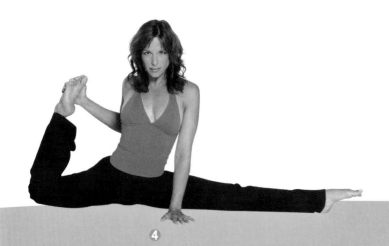

④

Chapter 5
Coordination

Coordination: *n.* harmonious adjustment or action, as of muscles in producing complex movements

What is there to say? Coordination is important? Well, that goes without saying. Outside of coordination being the one element that keeps you from bumping into walls, it's also the skill that most relates to physical aptitude. It's the main component for achieving superior athletic ability.

There are a lot of activities that really can challenge your coordination. Sports like tennis and racquetball are perfect: They combine timing, balance, and physical aptitude with mental awareness. All of these elements are necessary for simple daily functions. With the world being what it is today, everybody's multitasking all the time, which makes coordination that much more essential. Let's face it—these days life is all about efficiency.

Some people think you are born either clumsy or graceful, but that's simply not the case. Coordination is a skill that you can hone and practice and improve upon. My dance and martial arts classes were the perfect vehicles for mastering this particular skill. It came so easily to me because of the passion I had for these activities. Virtually any sport will help develop your coordination—so again, I encourage you to find what inspires you and go with it.

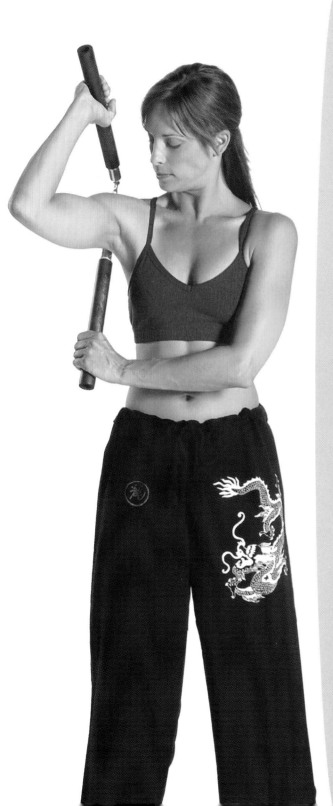

Your Inner Ear

Balance is a key component to good coordination. In any sport you participate in, being centered is essential. Anytime you're a little tired or sick, your equilibrium can be off and you have to work harder. Everything tends to slip out of whack.

Pressure can sometimes build up in your inner ear and cause dysfunction, which in turn affects your equilibrium. So here's a great little trick for when you're feeling off-center: Give a slight but quick downward tug to your earlobe at a 45-degree angle toward the floor (for children the tugging motion goes upward). This will release the pressure and reset your equilibrium.

Wanna Play?

Get in touch with your inner child and break out the toys! Some classic kids' games have withstood the test of time because they are fun *and* develop good coordination. Jacks, hopscotch, paddleball, and patty cake—these are all cool for gaining and maintaining basic hand-eye coordination.

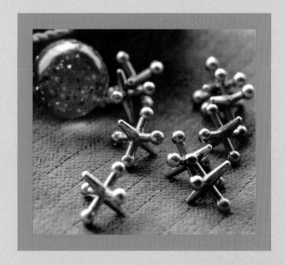

Timing Is Everything

There's not a stuntperson—or serious athlete, for that matter—who lacks coordination. It's simply something we cannot do without.

I would have to say that my biggest challenge in this regard was my job as Gear Girl on *Worst-Case Scenario*. For every episode we shot, I had to learn some new, off-the-wall, and dangerous activity. One thing always remained the same: There was never much time. I had two days to master the Jetboard, a motorized surfboard. The tricky thing was that I had to start the motor in the water and have perfect timing and balance to get the board going and stand up on it. Of course this went beyond simple operation of the equipment; I had to be able to carve turns and do all sorts of groovy tricks (after all, I *was* Gear Girl). This was not the easiest thing to do on a machine that went 40 miles an hour (64.3 kph), especially with obstacles like waves adding to the challenge.

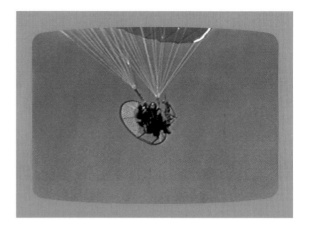

Then there was the motorized paraglider. I was actually lucky on this one—I had a full four days to practice on it. However, I was also dealing with a 10-pound (4.5 kg) motor on my back and a huge parachute that I had to learn to kite behind me. As I got everything perfectly lined up, I had to find just the right time to hit the throttle so that the motor could propel me into the air. Then there was the matter of climbing the machine high enough so I could land it on one of those giant rock formations that you see in Monument Valley, where the altitude is so high that the thin air makes it virtually impossible to fly.

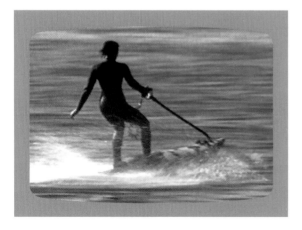

And last but not least, there's one of my favorites: the Gekkomat. This was a suction cup device that operated with an air compressor that attached to my back with hoses (the hoses ran to four paddles attached to my hands and feet). I was required to take the contraption up the side of a 26-story building, but because of some production complications, I had 20 minutes before the shoot to learn how to operate it. At the time, the machine was a prototype and had never been operated by a woman, nor had it ever scaled so high. To date, that was one of the scariest stunts of my career.

Obviously, these are extreme situations that you will probably never have to face, but I guarantee you that on any level, good coordination will make everything in your life smoother and more efficient. It really is the core of daily functioning. When your coordination is impaired, you may not be operating safely. Think about getting pulled over for a sobriety test. What do the state troopers check? Balance and coordination. So whether you want to perform better in your daily life or in your favorite sport or activity, developing these skills will be of great benefit.

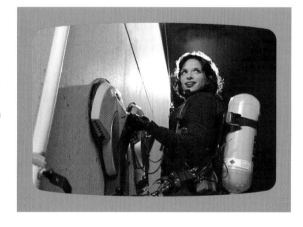

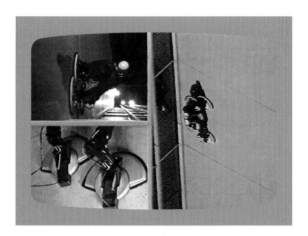

Air Time

I find my gymnastics training to be one of the most important skills I have in the stunt world. It gives you a sense of "air awareness," teaching you how to control your body in the air. Diving boards and trampolines are also great tools that provide you extra airtime to figure out the logistics of a trick, such as the backflip exercise you learned in Chapter 1 (page 70).

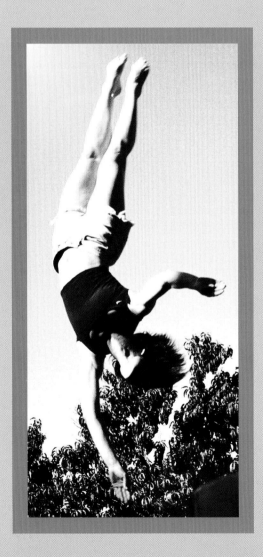

Coordination Exercises

Bruce Lee's favorite coordination exercise was playing Ping-Pong. Among fighters, a favorite exercise is working with a speed bag. Finding the coordination regimen that's right for you can be something as simple as finding the activity you enjoy the most. (Then of course there are other, more stationary activities that work your coordination—for example, playing a musical instrument.) All kinds of ball and racquet sports are great for developing hand-eye coordination (tennis, racquetball, squash, etc.). The common denominator here? Chasing a moving object.

Basic Balance

I use this exercise as a test to see where my balance is before doing something physical; but the simple act of doing it also has the added benefit of helping me center myself.

1. Start from a good standing position, feet hip-width apart. Stand strong and straight.

2. Close your eyes.

❸ Shift your weight to your left foot and raise your right foot just off the ground. Find your balance, keeping your body strong and straight.

4. Lower your right foot and shift your weight to it. Repeat the process by raising your left foot.

Variations:

● Once balanced, try rising up on the ball of your foot, remembering to keep your body tight. Your energy should be pushing into the ground while simultaneously lengthening toward the ceiling.

● To challenge yourself further, get creative with the non-weight-bearing leg. Put the bottom of your foot against the inside of your standing knee (as in Tree Pose, page 102) or hold your leg out out at a 90-degree angle from your body.

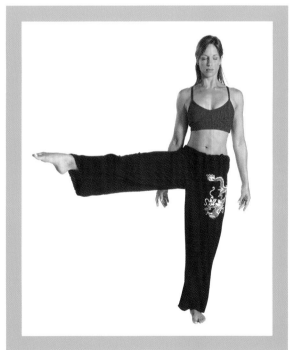

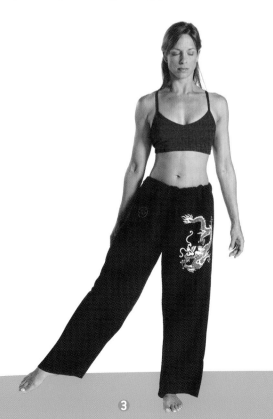

Martial Arts: Breaking It Down

There are more than 3,000 styles of martial arts, but they break down into two basic styles—hard and soft. The hard styles, which include karate, kickboxing, and tae kwan do, involve punching, kicking, and full-force attacks. They involve two bodies literally crashing into each other. These styles require explosive energy, overall strength, stamina, coordination, focus, and flexibility. In other words, they challenge you to become a phenomenal athlete.

And then there are the soft styles—tai chi, pau kua, and hsing-I. Their guiding principle is using the opponent's own energy against him/her by redirecting the attack without taking the blows. We call this parrying. (Refer to the "Trapping" exercise, page 107, for examples of parrying techniques.) Soft martial arts include self-defense techniques that many body types can master. They require focus and coordination above all else. Jujitsu and aikido are forms that combine both hard and soft styles.

Several other martial arts terms include:

- *Kung fu*, a general term for the combative arts.

- *Krav Maga*, an Israeli military combat form that incorporates several principles of martial arts.

- *Wu shu*, which originated in China after martial arts were outlawed by the Communist government. It takes on the appearance of a dance and has become one of the most graceful and fluid forms of fighting, hence its growing popularity in films such as *Crouching Tiger, Hidden Dragon*, *The Matrix*, and every Jet Li movie you've ever seen.

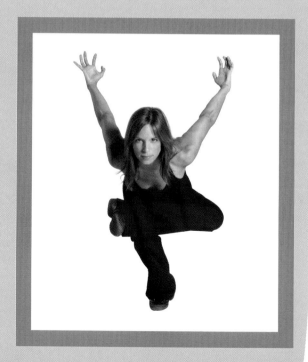

Coordination Exercises

Color Catch

Here's a simple hand-eye coordination exercise with a sprinkling of decision-making added to the mix to keep your mind sharp as a tack. You'll need a partner.

1. Grab some tennis balls and some markers. Create different colored balls—red, blue, green, orange and yellow. The more balls you can have in play, the better.

2. Delegate which ball represents which reaction. For example, always catch the red ball with the right hand, the blue ball with the left hand; dodge the green ball to the right, and dodge the yellow ball to the left.

3. There are no rules for beginning the exercise. One person can start with all the balls and throw them at his partner, or you can each throw balls at the same time. Every time the exercise starts over, change it up.

4. Feel free to get creative: Make up new responses and change the speed of the exercise. If you like, you can devise a basic scorekeeping system.

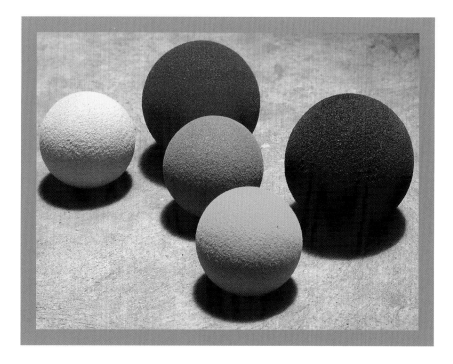

Juggling is probably one of the best hand-eye coordination drills you can do. Once you master it, it's a great party trick to pull out of your bag. (It might even inspire you to run off and join the circus!)

A note about choosing balls: The heavier the ball, the easier the exercise. Lacrosse balls work well, as do rubber dog balls. Beanbags are also excellent for learning—they don't roll away when you drop them.

With two balls (called a circle):

① Start with two balls in one hand. You will be working with one hand only for this exercise. I recommend that you start out with your dominant hand. Your arm should be at an approximate right angle, elbow close to the body, forearm out in front.

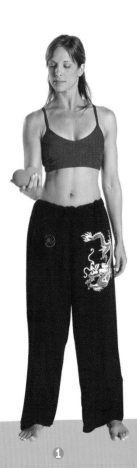

①

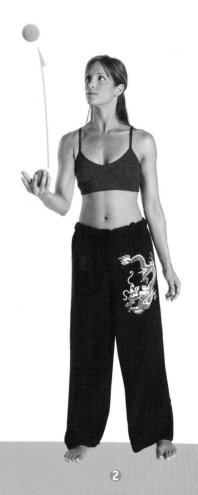

②

2 Throw ball 1 in the air, giving it a slight inside arc. You will be making a circle, inside to outside. Keep the ball within eye level and don't let it go too far to the right or the left.

3 Just before ball 1 makes it back to your hand, release ball 2 into the air. It's all about the timing here, and you will find that it's better to throw late.

4 Catch ball 1 with the same hand, while ball 2 is at the top of its arc.

5. Repeat steps 2 to 4 for as many rounds as you can keep the balls in the air.

Variations:
Once you master your dominant hand, practice with your non-dominant hand. Then work both hands simultaneously.

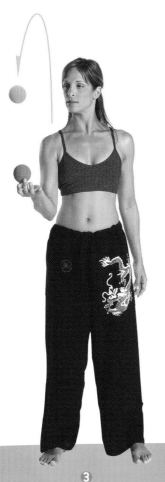

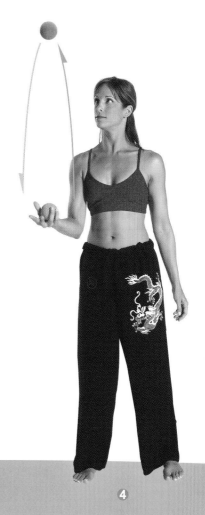

3

4

With three balls (called a cascade):

1 Start with two balls in your dominant hand, one ball in your opposite hand.

2. The throwing motion here is going to be underhanded, and the balls will be moving inside to outside, creating a figure 8 in front of you. Again, remember: It's all about the timing, and it's better to throw at the last second.

3 Throw ball 1 with your dominant hand. Keep your balls in range and within eye level.

4. Throw ball 2 with your non-dominant hand.

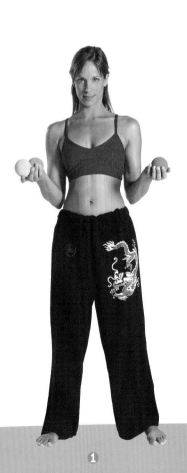

1

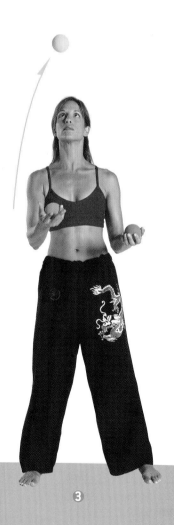

3

⑤ Catch ball 1 with your non-dominant hand.

6. Throw ball 3 with your dominant hand.

⑦ Catch ball 2 with your dominant hand. Continue the figure-8 motion.

Mastering this skill takes a good amount of practice. And it's great for exercising your patience as well as your coordination.

Variations:

- To make things easier on yourself, you can slow the motion of the balls by practicing underwater in a swimming pool.

- Once you've mastered the basics, go to town. Multiply the number of balls you use or move up to rings, clubs, objects on fire, and the like.

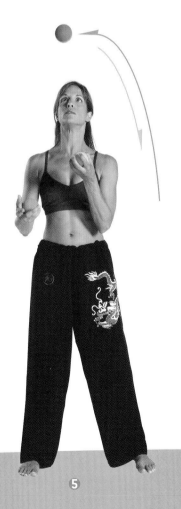

5

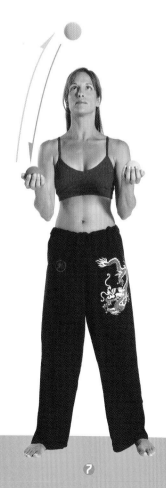

7

Coordination Exercises

Nunchaku

A nunchaku is a weapon consisting of two thick sticks joined at their ends by a rawhide band, rope, or chain. However, martial arts supply stores sell rubber versions that are effective tools for building dexterity. Here's a really basic drill. From here, the sky's the limit.

❶ Hold one stick in your right hand with your elbow close to your side and your arm starting at a 90-degree angle.

❷ Swing the second stick up and back so that it ends up behind your right shoulder blade. As it completes its rotation, grab hold of the second stick with your left hand by reaching in front of you, under your right armpit.

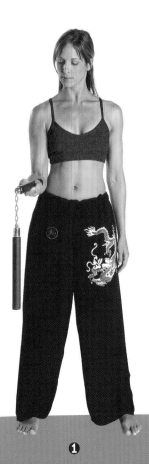

❶

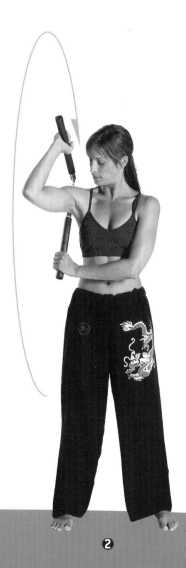

❷

❸ Release your right grip and allow that end to swing up and over your left shoulder.

❹ As the stick reaches behind your left shoulder blade, grab it with your right hand.

5. Repeat the process, continuing with fluid movement.

Variation:

• Once you've mastered this basic technique, I encourage you to learn more complicated moves from an instructor or a video. It will really challenge your coordination and benefit your focus—not to mention, it's fun and makes you look like Bruce Lee!

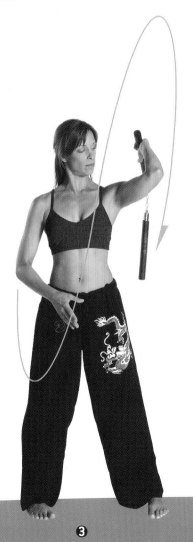

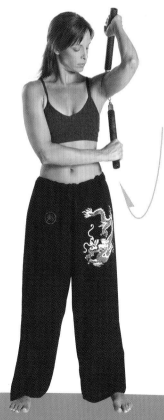

❸

❹

Chapter 6
Speed

Speed: *n.* the act or state of moving rapidly; swiftness; quick motion

I find that, in general, people don't think speed is an important attribute to have in their adult lives. After training for wind sprints in junior high, we just don't really give any weight to speed training. But the reality is that there are great benefits to being quick on your feet.

Speed is about more than just outrunning the Road Runner. It's the ability to have explosive energy. For boxers, it's the element of bobbing, weaving, and throwing a knockout punch that comes out of nowhere. It's the basketball player's vertical jump. It's the gymnast's takeoff to complete a double twist. It's the runner's blast out of the starting blocks.

Get the picture? When I'm talking about speed, I mean more than running from point A to point B in a short amount of time. I'm talking about those bursts of high energy that all athletes need. Which brings me to the topic of fast-twitch muscles.

Your muscles are broken up into slow- and fast-twitch muscle fibers that are distributed throughout your body. Fast-twitch muscles are responsible for explosive strength, and slow-twitch ones are for controlled strength and endurance. You also have muscle fibers that are middle of the road and can go either way. When you do plyometrics (explosive power training), you convert the medium muscle fibers into fast-twitch. This fast-twitch muscle fiber is very dense, so you can't have a whole body full of it.

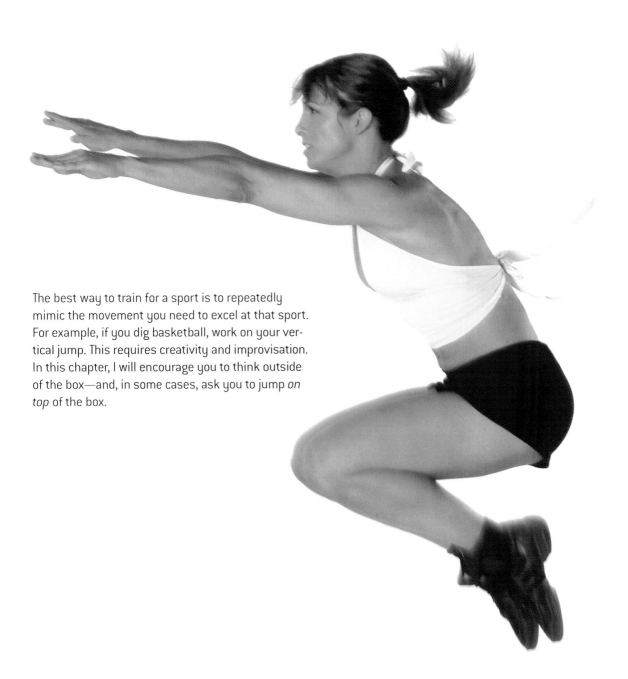

The best way to train for a sport is to repeatedly mimic the movement you need to excel at that sport. For example, if you dig basketball, work on your vertical jump. This requires creativity and improvisation. In this chapter, I will encourage you to think outside of the box—and, in some cases, ask you to jump *on top* of the box.

The Need for Speed

There are two main factors for determining your progress when training for speed: how high you jump from a standing position and how fast you run a short distance. However, depending on your sport, there may be other ways to gauge your speed. (For example, boxers are going to be more concerned with hand speed.) It doesn't matter what you're attempting to do, however: If you need more speed, you need a massive force of explosive ability.

For my film work, I am constantly called upon to get creative and to train specifically for a required stunt. While shooting an episode of the action TV series *Martial Law*, I had to leap across the width of a rooftop pool. There was no space for a running start, so I relied on my fast-twitch muscles to explode off one side of the pool and still cover the distance. I mapped the space out in my backyard and repeatedly worked the stunt until I felt confident that I would clear the edge. I had three close calls but never fell in!

In action films, it's always important to look explosive. Jackie Chan is my hero because he's got the market cornered on dynamic fight sequences. He certainly demonstrates the need to get out of the way if something is hurtling toward your head. And if you've ever watched his outtakes, you can see why it's so critical that he be quick on his feet.

Speaking of objects flying at your head brings to mind *Dodgeball: A True Underdogs Story*. During rehearsals for the dodgeball games in the movie, I was hired to be the target for pro volleyball players, who whizzed the ball at me as hard and fast as they could. So let me reiterate: Speed is important. Lack of speed may result in pain and humiliation.

Aside from these extreme examples, I hope you're beginning to see why speed counts when engaging both in physical activity and in everyday life. Speed is a key factor in helping you become a phenomenal athlete, because in combination with strength, it results in incredible power.

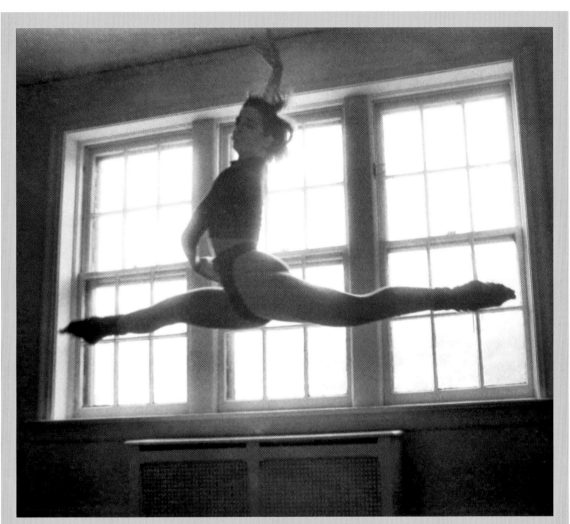

Explosive power is vital in many sports, including dance.

These exercises are designed to shock the muscles. They are strenuous and violent movements, so you'd better seriously warm up. Give your body a good day or two of rest between these workouts, because they tax the body. You may not hit failure, but you'll exhaust yourself. Don't push yourself too hard at the outset.

Levels: 1–5

This is probably the most basic speed exercise. You might remember it from your junior high gym class. Be sure to wear a good pair of running shoes.

1. Set yourself a point A and a point B. The distance between the two points should be short, certainly no more than 50 yards (45.7 m).

❷ At point A, assume a good takeoff position. Pitch slightly over your knees, with your back straight. Bend from the waist so that you're leaning at a 45-degree angle. Place your dominant foot forward, making sure your knee is in line with your foot. Your other foot should be slightly behind you. You should be on the balls of your feet.

Takeoff position at point A.

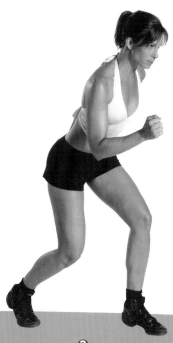

❷

❸ Remember, what we are training for here is explosive energy, so on the takeoff, push off as hard as you can.

❹ Keeping your weight slightly forward and arms pumping close to your body, run fast and hard to point B.

5. Before you repeat this exercise, rest until your pulse drops to a near-normal rate.

Try to achieve five reps. The stronger you get, the more you should increase your distance and reps. You can also do this on an incline for a further challenge.

Push off with explosive energy.

Run fast and hard to point B.

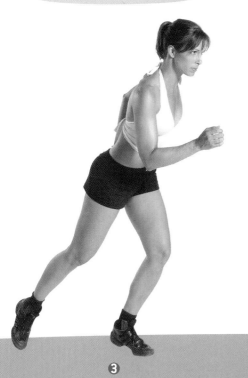

❸

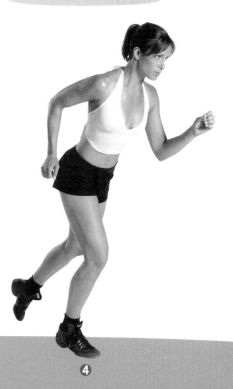

❹

Hip Hop Hooray

Levels: 1–5

Here's another great basic power drill that builds overall explosive leg strength, specifically in the glutes, hamstrings, and quads.

1. Start with your knees slightly bent, a straight back, and arms by your sides.

2. Keeping your head up, jump as high as you can, forcefully bringing your arms straight up for additional lift.

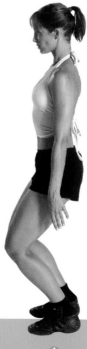

1

❸ At the height of the jump, fully extend your body.

❹ As you land, bend your knees so that you end in the same position as you began.

5. Repeat 10 times; as you get stronger, increase the number of sets, making sure to rest a few minutes between each one.

Tip:
Measure your progress by doing this exercise alongside a wall. Either put chalk on your fingers or grab hold of a piece of tape. At the height of your jump, mark the wall.

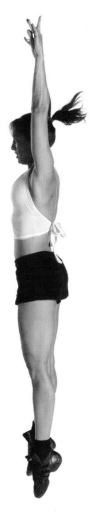

3

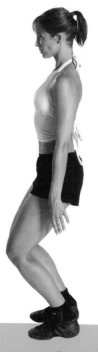

4

Box Hop

Levels: 2–5

This advanced version of Hip Hop Hooray requires one sturdy box or table between 1 and 2 feet (0.3–0.6 m) high. This platform should support your weight and not slide around. I love to do these on apple boxes, since they are always lying around film sets and come in a variety of heights. When I'm doing stunts on set and I have to do a stunt off an apple box, I pack sand bags around it to prevent it from sliding.

❶ Stand about 2 to 3 steps away from the box. Face the box and start in the same position as Hip Hop Hooray.

❷ Keeping your head up, jump forward and as high as you can, forcefully bringing your arms straight out for additional lift.

❸ Land in the center of the box, bending your knees slightly to absorb the impact. Safely hop back down and repeat.

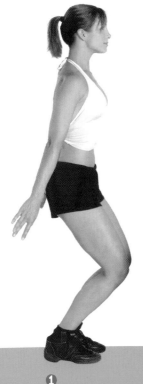
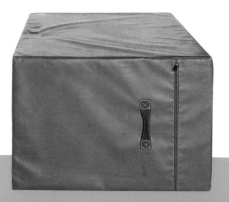

❶

Do no more than 10 reps in a set. The better you get, the more sets you can do.

Tip:

If you're really challenging yourself, chances are you might not clear the box. Always be ready to use your hands to either assist or protect you. If you're concerned about safety, you can also place mats around the box.

Variation:

- For a more advanced variation, find an even higher, stable box. Take a slight running start, and punch off the ground from both feet, driving your knees up toward your chest so your feet clear the box.

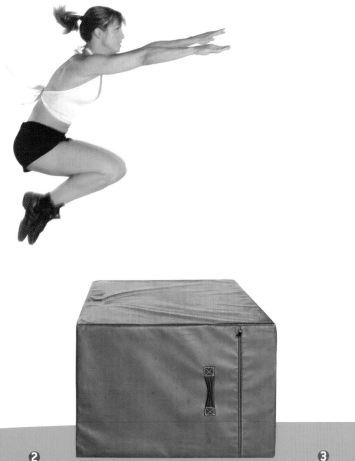

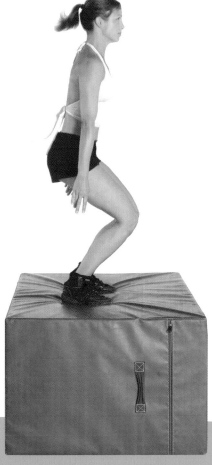

❷

❸

Zig Zags

Levels: 2–5

This is a great exercise for lateral movement and explosive leg strength.

You'll need an obstacle to jump over. The height of the obstacle will depend on your level of expertise. Ideally, you want to build up to a 2-foot (0.6 m) high jump, so start with an object anywhere between 1 and 2 feet (0.3–0.6 m) high. This exercise is traditionally done with cones, but you can use anything at your preferred height, such as a stack of books. Set the two cones 2 to 3 feet (0.6–0.9 m) apart.

❶ Stand with your feet facing forward to the right of both cones. You will remain facing forward throughout this exercise.

❷ Jump to your left over the first cone, driving your knees up and pumping your arms to help your lift and balance.

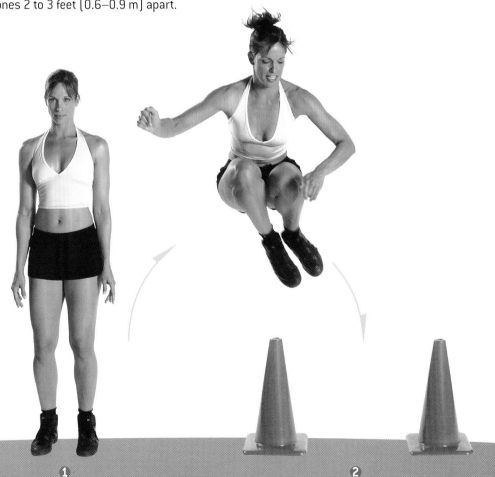

❶   ❷

❸ Land in the center of the two cones.

❹ *Immediately* jump left again over the second cone in the same manner.

5. Jump back to the center without hesitating and then back again to the right over the first cone.

6. Do 5 reps per set, and rest a couple of minutes between each set. As you get faster and stronger, increase the number of sets.

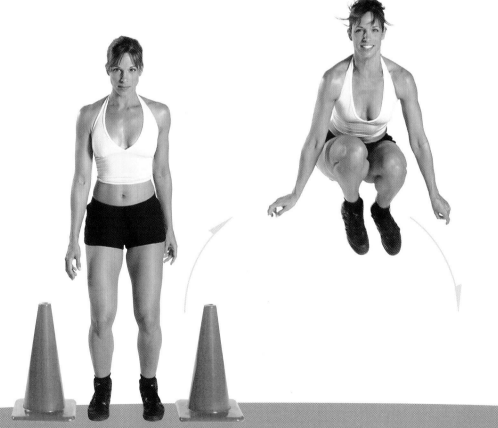

❸

❹

These two exercises develop explosive upper body and arm strength. Try for 10 reps per set, and rest a couple of minutes between each set. As you get faster and stronger, increase your sets.

Heavy Bag
Levels: 1–5

You need a hanging heavy bag for this exercise. You can usually find one at the gym or your local sporting goods store.

① Assume a comfortable stance, left foot slightly forward, with your right arm at a right angle to your body and your fist placed lightly against the heavy bag.

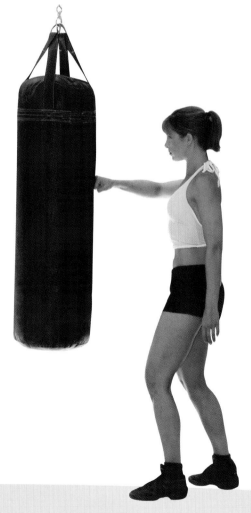

①

2. With one explosive motion, fully extend your right arm and use your body weight to push the bag. As your arm extends forward, move your left shoulder back, allowing your torso to twist. Continue the action until the bag swings away from the body.

3. Catch the bag on its return.

4. Work both arms, one at a time, repeating to exhaustion.

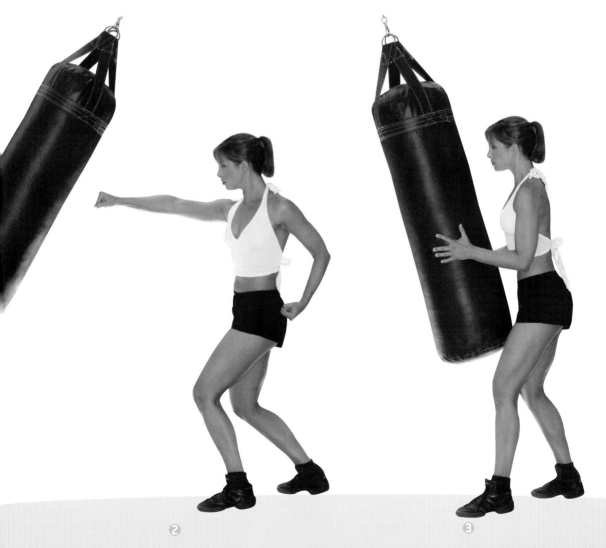

Medicine Ball

Levels: 3–5

You'll need a 9- to 16-pound (4–7.2 kg) medicine ball for this exercise. You may want to do this outside in a flat area, and you may want to invite a friend to help retrieve the ball as well as measure your distance. *Don't* expect your partner to catch it—medicine balls pack a dangerous punch.

❶ Start from a good standing position, knees slightly bent, feet hip-width apart, and back straight. With your arms bent, hold the ball against your chest.

❷ With one explosive motion, extend your arms, throwing the ball out and as far as possible. Keeping your body tight and strong will prevent you from pitching forward.

3. Measure your progress by measuring the distance of your throw.

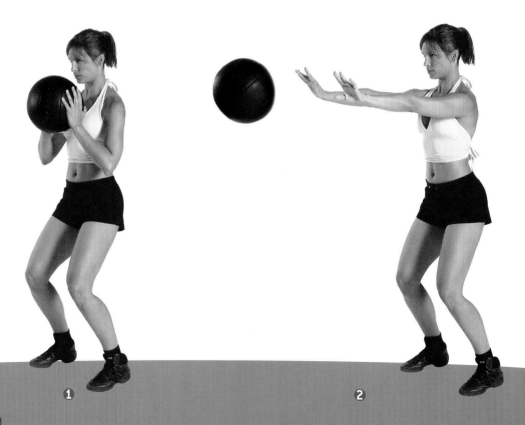

1. Start by kneeling on a soft surface, with your toes curled under. Hold the ball with both hands behind your head, with arms slightly bent.

2. Lean back slightly, and then quickly and powerfully throw the ball by leaning forward and extending your arms out in front of you.

3. Once you release the ball, allow your body to continue forward until your hands hit the ground.

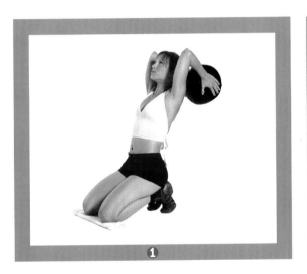

1

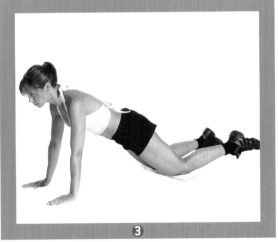

3

Chapter 7
The Circuits

Circuit: *n.* 1 a complete round of exercises 2 the regular journey of a person performing certain tasks

Okay, people, this is where it all comes together. I hope that if you've learned anything from this book, it's the fact that your personal passion should be what dictates your physical activity. I want you to take on a new mental outlook and allow that new passion to trigger a healthy change in your life. Too many people make the effort to get fit or lose weight by trying fad workouts and diets. The results are almost always temporary. But if you find an activity that feeds your soul, you will stay healthy and happy forever.

As I've mentioned throughout this book, it's important to remember to challenge yourself, but if it's your passion that's fueling you, your progression will naturally take care of itself. Without that inner drive, people tend to become bored or lose their inspiration and therefore become complacent in their workouts. Then they wonder why they're not getting stronger or thinner. Pay attention to whether you're maintaining or making progress. At the same time, don't be too hard on yourself. Some days you're just *off*. It simply may not be your day, no matter what sport you're doing. Realize that it's just a moment in time and a part of the process. Don't give up.

The circuits that follow are combinations of exercises that incorporate many of the skills featured throughout this book. However, I'm firm in my belief that you will be more inclined to stick with your fitness regimen if you also get your workout through the sports that you love. For example, if you're into rock climbing, go climb that rock! You are going to be working your strength, endurance, focus, coordination, and flexibility. In other words, you will be embarking on a wonderfully challenging circuit. Train according to your passion—customize your circuit workout depending on the sport in which you're interested (see chart on pages 16–17).

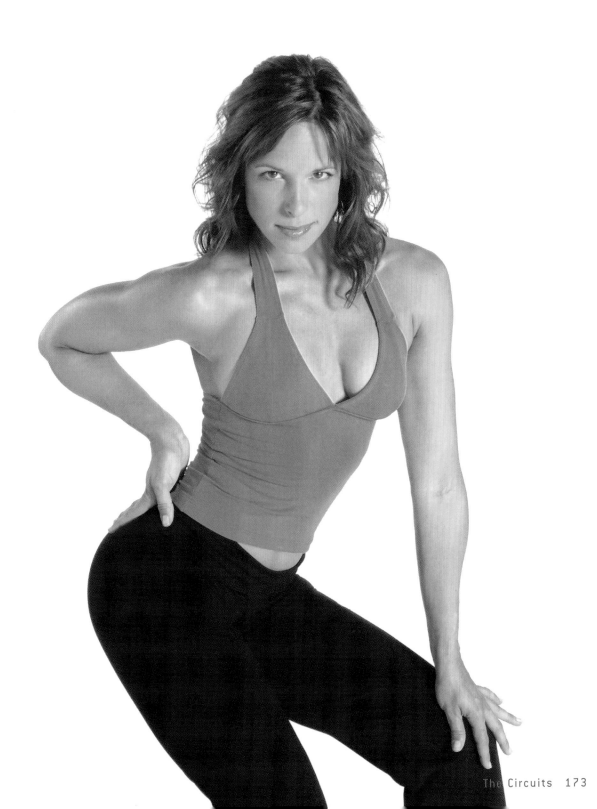

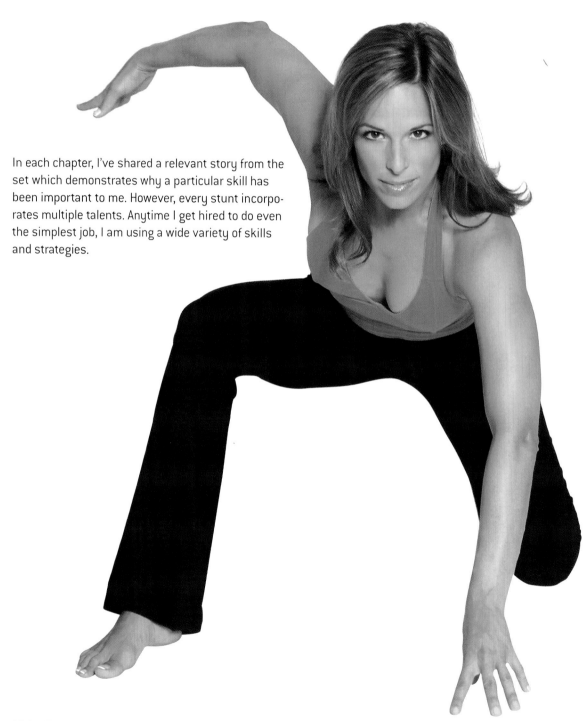

Putting It Together

In each chapter, I've shared a relevant story from the set which demonstrates why a particular skill has been important to me. However, every stunt incorporates multiple talents. Anytime I get hired to do even the simplest job, I am using a wide variety of skills and strategies.

By now, you probably have a good grip on my personal passions, and so you know how much I love to fight. My absolute favorite brawl was with Tiffani Thiessen in a prison yard on *Fastlane*. It was a brutal girl fight that tested my strength, endurance, focus, coordination, flexibility, and speed. Overall strength came in handy for those fierce kicks and punches; it also helped protect my bones when she flipped me onto the hard ground. I needed the endurance to get through take after take of high-energy fighting. My concentration was taxed from remembering the fight choreography and staying alert to everything going on around me. (When fists are flying by your head and you're flinging your body within inches of a camera, you'd best be focused.) I think the coordination factor speaks for itself—there were several intricate moves to the fight, and if we got out of sync with each other, someone could have seriously gotten hurt. My flexibility training came into play, as I had to contort my body to "sell" the violence as believable. And last but not least, speed was necessary to make it all look powerful and dynamic.

I'm not encouraging you to train for catfights, but I do want you to understand the importance of a full spectrum of exercise. The circuits that follow are simply suggestions to get you started. From there, I want you to come up with your own routine.

I can't say it enough: Everyone is different. Only you know what works best for you.

This, finally, is what my book has been about. Find what moves you—literally and figuratively!

Solar Power

When the weather's nice, try doing the exercises in this book outside to change things up. Treat your body to fresh air, sun, and the stimuli around you. Outdoor activity is an amazing gift, and you should indulge in it.

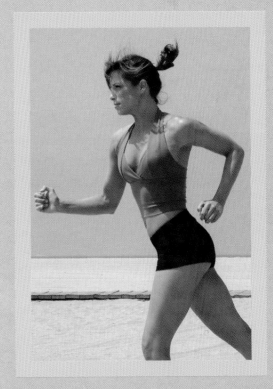

The Circuits

These circuits have been set up to work different body parts on different days. It's important to allow muscles to recuperate sufficiently between work-outs for optimal efficiency. Five days of good training per week is plenty. You get to decide where to incorporate your two days off.

Make up your own circuits. For example, when it comes to cardio/endurance, you can shadowbox (page 83). For speed, you can do three 3-minute rounds on the heavy bag (page 168). Get creative before you get bored. Or scrap circuits altogether and go play a game of tennis!

This circuit program is a good, basic formula for all-around fitness. If it's too challenging, ease your way into it. If it's not challenging enough, substitute more advanced exercises from the preceding sections.

Day 1

These exercises are best done with a partner and primarily work coordination, endurance, and focus. If you don't have someone to team up with, substitute another coordination and cardio activity combination today. Pick exercises from Chapters 2 and 5 that appeal to you the most (or pick an activity from the "Picking Your Passion" chart on pages 16–17).

This circuit is a fun, light workout that will hone your focus and coordination.

Warm-up: Roll It Out and Stretches 1–4 (page 22)

Coordination: Color Catch (page 149)

Endurance/Cardio: Follow the Leader (20 minutes) (page 88)

Focus:
1. Mirror Image (page 106)
2. Trapping (page 107)

Cool-down (same as warm-up) (page 22)

Warm-up

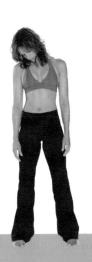

Color Catch

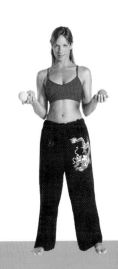

Follow the Leader

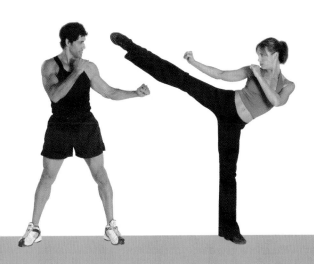

Mirror Image

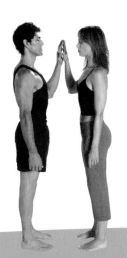

Trapping

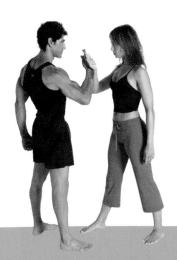

Cool-down

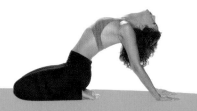

Combined, these exercises focus on your foundation by working your legs and abdominal muscles as well as strengthening your heart. You'll end with a series of flexibility stretches to cool down.

Warm-up: Roll It Out and Stretches 1–4 (page 22)

Endurance/Cardio: Bleacher Blastoff (20 minutes) (page 85)

Strengthening:
1. Legs: Oldie but Goodie Squats (3 sets) (page 44)
2. Legs: Basic Lunges (3 sets) (page 46)
3. Legs: Rise and Shine (3 sets) (page 48)
4. Abs: Standard Issue Sit-ups (go to failure) (page 64)
5. Abs: The Twist (go to failure) (page 66)

Flexibility:
1. Hip Stretch 1 (page 120)
2. Thigh Stretch 1 (page 126)
3. Hamstring Stretch 1 (page 133)

| Warm-up | Bleacher Blastoff | Oldie but Goodie Squats | Basic Lunges |

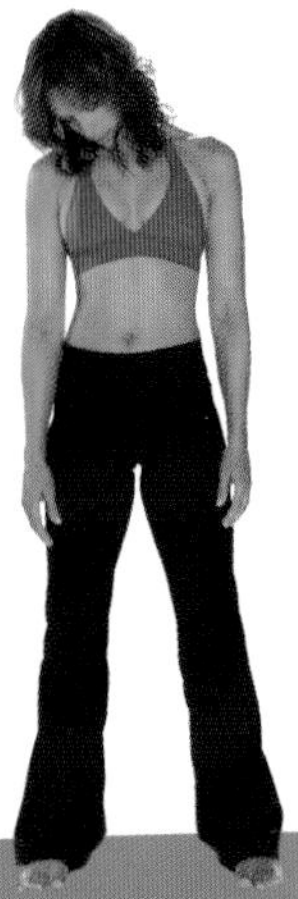

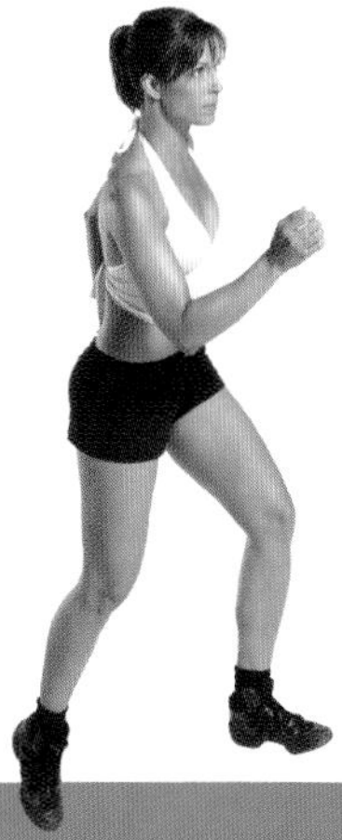

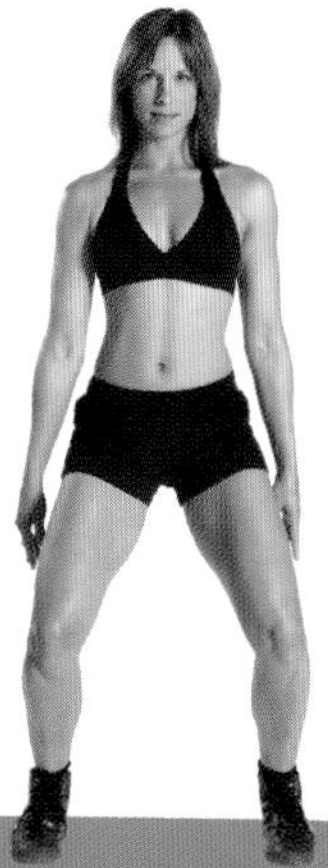

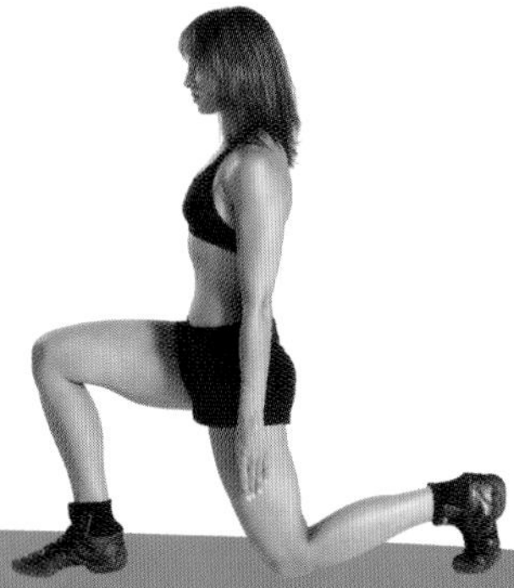

Rise and Shine

Standard Issue Sit-ups

The Twist

Hip Stretch 1

Thigh Stretch 1

Hamstring Stretch 1

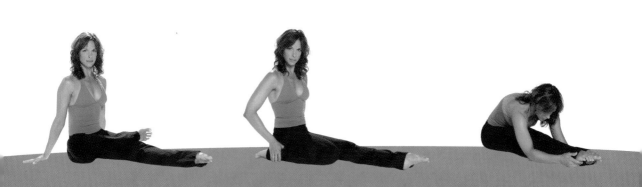

Basically, this day is all about "pulling" strength. Remember that muscle groups should be worked together and be given proper recovery time, except, of course, for your quick-healing abs. (You may want to integrate one abdominal exercise into each day's circuit, if your energy is high.) Start this workout with some good music and keep your groove on through the circuit. Cool down with two basic flexibility stretches.

Warm-up: Roll It Out and Stretches 1–4 (page 22)

Endurance/Cardio: Get Your Groove On (20 minutes) (page 84)

Strengthening:
1. Back/Biceps: Classic Chin-ups/Pull-ups (Advanced) (3 sets) (page 50)
2. Back/Biceps: The Bend and Stand (3 sets) (page 54)
3. Back/Biceps: Bulging Bicep Curls (3 sets) (page 55)
4. Abs: Standard Issue Sit-ups (go to failure) (page 64)

Flexibility:
1. Back Stretch 3 (page 132)
2. Glute Stretch 1 (page 128)

Warm-up

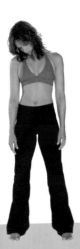

Get Your Groove On

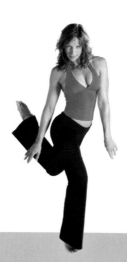

Chin-ups/Pull-ups

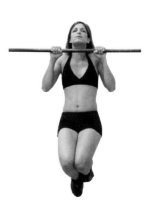

The Bend and Stand

Bulging Bicep Curls

Standard Issue Sit-ups

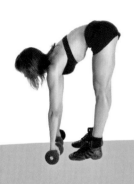

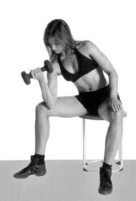

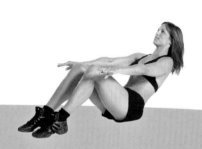

Back Stretch 3

Glute Stretch 1

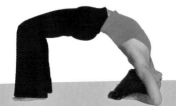

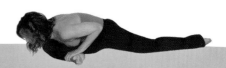

Day 4

You guessed it—today is all about "pushing" strength. To keep the workout lively, I've thrown in an outdoor cardio activity that will work your creativity as well as your heart. Let the great outdoors energize you and help you through the rest of this challenging circuit.

Warm-up: Roll It Out and Stretches 1–4 (page 22)

Flexibility: Shoulder Stretch 2 (page 118)

Endurance/Cardio: Create Your Own Course (20 minutes) (page 87)

Strengthening:
1. Chest/Shoulders/Triceps: Old School Push-ups (3 sets) (page 56)
2. Chest/Shoulders/Triceps: Handstand Push-ups (3 sets) (page 59)
3. Chest/Shoulders/Triceps: The Dip (3 sets) (page 62)
4. Abs: The Twist (go to failure) (page 66)

Cool-down (same as warm-up) (page 22)

| Warm-up | Shoulder Stretch 2 | Create Your Own Course |

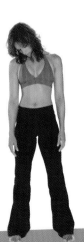
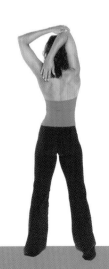
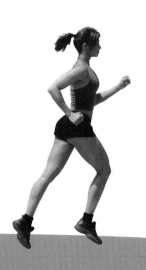

Old School Push-ups

Handstand Push-ups

The Dip

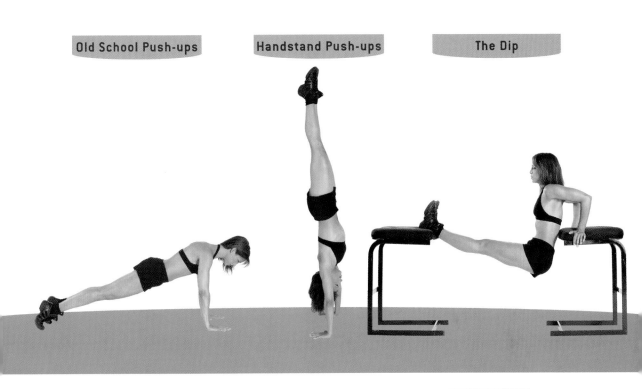

The Twist

Cool-down

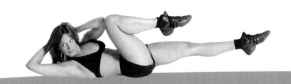

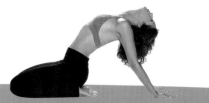

At first blush, this seems like a really ambitious circuit. And it is. But I think this is one of the most rewarding workouts. The flexibility exercises will feel great and get you primed and ready for the speed exercises, which are powerful but playful.

Warm-up: Roll It Out and Stretches 1–4 (page 22)

Flexibility:
1. Shoulder Stretch 1 (page 116)
2. Hip Stretch 2 (page 122)
3. Thigh Stretch 1 (page 126)
4. Glute Stretch 1 (page 128)
5. Back Stretch 2 (page 131)
6. Hamstring Stretch 2 (page 135)
7. Inner Thigh Stretch 1 (page 136)

Speed:
1. Speed Demon Sprints (5 sets) (page 160)
2. Hip Hop Hooray (10 reps/set, 3 sets) (page 162)
3. Zig Zags (5 reps/set, 3 sets) (page 166)

Cool-down (same as warm-up) (page 22)

Warm-up	Shoulder Stretch 1	Hip Stretch 2	Thigh Stretch 1

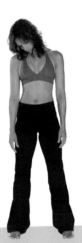
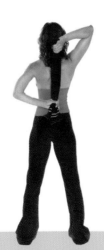
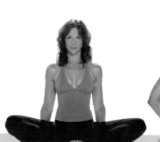
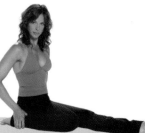

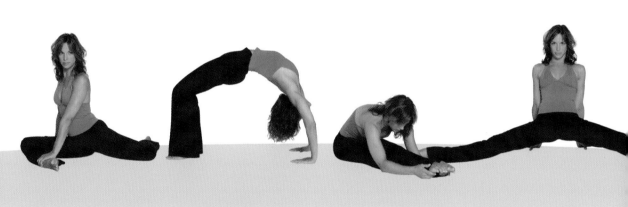

Glute Stretch 1   Back Stretch 2   Hamstring Stretch 2   Inner Thigh Stretch 1

Speed Demon Sprints   Hip Hop Hooray   Zig Zags   Cool-down

The Stuntwoman's Glossary

Here are some terms mentioned in the book that I wanted to further define. Just for fun, I threw in some stunt terms so that you can expand your knowledge of the magic of movie making. It goes without saying, of course, that stunt work should be performed only by skilled professionals.

Air ram
A pneumatic device that catapults you through the air through the use of intense air pressure. The force of an air ram can range anywhere from a few hundred pounds to more than a thousand pounds of pressure.

BASE jumping
Free falling off a stationary object with the use of a parachute for landing. BASE stands for Building, Antennae, Span, Earth, and represents the fixed objects from which BASE jumps are made.

Breakaway
Chairs, bottles, or any props that are specially designed by the FX department to easily and safely shatter upon contact.

Calisthenics
Exercises, such as sit-ups and push-ups, that use your own body weight to develop a strong, trim physique.

Candied glass
Created to simulate glass objects or surfaces in many films for safety purposes, this material is made from a sugar-based substance that breaks easily.

Cannon roll
A car stunt that is performed when a cylindrical object is shot out of the bottom of a car, causing the car to roll or flip.

Cortisol
A steroid hormone secreted by the adrenal glands, important in stress response and in regulating blood sugar and fat deposition.

Electrolytes
Magnesium, potassium, phosphorus, and other elements that help keep your body hydrated. Sports drinks are designed to replenish your electrolyte level.

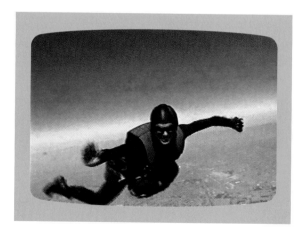

Endorphins
Any of several peptides secreted in the brain that have a pain-relieving effect like that of morphine.

Face-off
One of the main techniques for jumping off a building. You fall face down and do a half-twist at the last second so that you land on your back.

Gainer

A gymnastics move used in films, it is essentially a backflip that travels forward; it can be tucked or open. High divers love this move.

Header

One of the main techniques for jumping off a building. You fall face down and half somersault at the last second to land on your back.

Krav Maga

A form of self-defense created by the Israeli military which specializes in practical hand-to-hand combat techniques.

Kung fu

A general term for many Chinese martial arts.

Lactic acid

If you work out for too long and become dehydrated, your muscles start gasping for nutrition. Your body produces lactic acid, and the result is a burning sensation or shaky muscle.

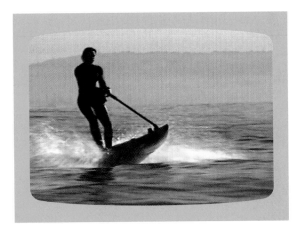

Nomex

Fire-retardant material that stuntpeople wear for fire protection or during fire stunts.

Nunchaku

A martial arts weapon consisting of two thick sticks joined at their ends by a rawhide band, rope, or chain.

Parrying

The deflection of a kick or a punch being thrown at you.

Pipe ramp

A car stunt that involves a car hitting a pipe or piece of steel at a particular angle and length, which causes the car to go airborne and twist in mid-air.

Plyometrics

An exercise technique to develop power by training both speed and strength simultaneously. The result is an increase in fast-twitch muscle fiber.

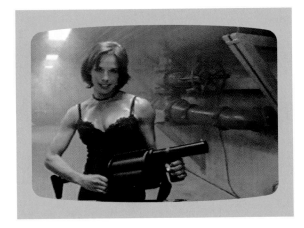

Port-a-Pit
A very large, thick pad used to catch stuntpeople after they've jumped off buildings and other heights.

Ratchet
A stunt whereby a person is attached to a line and violently jerked through the air by the use of high-speed hydraulics (for example, when thrown by King Kong or kicked by Catwoman).

Sliding 90s
When a stunt driver in a car chase purposely loses traction around a corner so that the car fishtails.

Span sets
A reinforced type of webbing used by stunt riggers to secure shivs (pulleys) for wire stunts. We use this when a stunt calls for a huge amount of force on the line (e.g., someone flying forward and then getting jerked backward).

Spotter
A sports professional who stands nearby to assist you, if necessary, when you are learning a stunt or gymnastics trick.

Squib
Mini-explosives that are often used to simulate a gunshot.

Stunt double
A specially trained performer who actually does stunts in place of a principal actor.

Tempered glass
Glass that is heated to a specific temperature to explode into very small, safe pieces with the help of squibs. When attempting to dive through this glass on a movie set, timing is imperative, since you make contact with the glass just as it blows. If you don't time it right, you may bounce off the glass or knock yourself out, which is very embarrassing and painful.

Webbing
This particular material—a thin, flat, strong strap—was originally used by rock climbers for just about everything. In stunts, we use webbing for both tying off shivs (pulleys) and constructing makeshift harnesses that are easily concealed under wardrobe. It's an old-school alternative to harnesses and is still widely used in Hong Kong films.

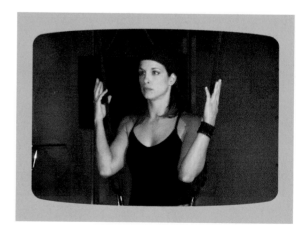

Index

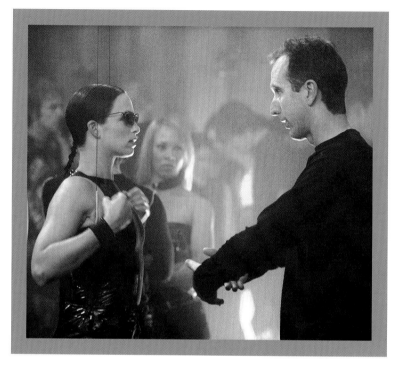

Acknowledgments

I want to take a minute to tell you about the following people, who not only helped me gather information for this book, but have been a huge source of learning, support, and friendship in my life. You may notice that the majority are men. Yeah, I'm a woman living in a man's world, and it's not a bad place to be!

Damian Achilles has spent years as a celebrity physical trainer, competitive bodybuilder, and manager of one of the most prestigious gyms in New York City. He also happens to be an incredible artist and friend, and I want to thank him for making me look so good in the photos throughout this book.

Sergio Carbajal has an extensive career incorporating many physical skills. Always on the lookout for a new physical passion, he started as a dancer and is a phenomenal gymnast, martial artist, and football player.

Joe Carey graduated from USC Medical School with high honors. He has a master's in anatomy and neurobiology.

Mitch Gould is my training partner and fellow stuntperson. His credits include *Ultraviolet*, *The Rundown*, *Wild Wild West*, and many more. An expert in martial arts techniques, he was hired as Lucy Liu's trainer on *Ballistic: Ecks vs. Severs*.

Jeff Imada is one of Hollywood's most famous stunt coordinators, the one who gave me my big break. He has coordinated many wonderful films, including *The Bourne Supremacy* (fight coordinator), *8 Mile*, *Daredevil*, *L.A. Confidential*, and *The Crow*. He's recognizable in front of the screen as well, with acting roles in blockbusters such as *Payback*, *Lethal Weapon 4*, *Escape from L.A.*, and *Big Trouble in Little China*.

Dan Southworth is a wonderful actor and stuntman, with credits including *The Tuxedo*, *Scorpion King*, and *The Rundown*.

Theo VanLondersele and Ji Lee are my chiropractors at Back in Action in Studio City, California. They are passionate about their work and about promoting greater understanding of the human body.

Mike Washlake is my gymnastics coach and a veteran stuntman with credits ranging from *Blade Runner* to *Scorpion King* and many others in between, including *Big Trouble in Little China*, *Spaceballs*, *Hook*, *Face/Off*, *Bowfinger*, and *Pearl Harbor*.

And then there's Jennifer Worick, the one and only, who has been with me every bump and turn on this incredible new adventure in writing. At the beginning of this process we barely knew each other, but she held my hand, guided me through, and filled the hours with support and laughter. It wasn't always easy, but because of what I learned about myself through her, it was always a pleasure. Now, at the end of the journey, I have a lifelong friend.

I'd also like to thank the following: Mom, Dad, and Tara for being my undying source of support; Carl Scott and Jon Simmons of Simmons and Scott Entertainment, along with my amazing management team of Cary, Shepard, and Don; Peter Bergmann; Gina McKenzie; Ed Zimmerman; Bob Garrigus; John Carpenter; Joel Silver; Roman Culjat; Alisse Kingsley and Stephanie Figura at Muse Media; all of my new friends at Quirk; and last but not least, Les Sheldon, someone whom I've always wanted to have lunch with. Thanks to all of my incredible family and friends, who are always there for me on so many levels. You all make my life rich.

About the Authors

Danielle Burgio, one of Hollywood's top stunt-women, has appeared in many blockbuster films, worked alongside some of the world's biggest celebrities, and experienced adventure that most of us only dream of. From diving through windows to scaling high-rise buildings with suction cups, Danielle has done it all—and has loved every minute of it. Along the way she has trained with some of the industry's top athletes and quickly adopted the "Go big or go home" credo that the stunt community lives by. Through her years of experience she has learned to focus on her goals, face her fears, and follow her passion through her personal philosophy and regimen for a healthy, happy, and active life-style. When not on location, Danielle lives in Sherman Oaks, California, with her dog, Harley.

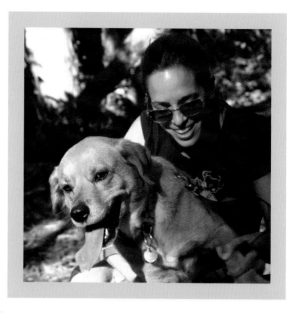

Her stunt credits include:

Angel	Ghosts of Mars	Not Another Teen Movie
Batman Forever	The Green Mile	Pearl Harbor
Birds of Prey	Helter Skelter	Power Rangers
Blade	Hollywood Homicide	Spanglish
Cellular	John Carpenter's Vampires	Summer of Sam
Charmed	Little Nicky	Will & Grace
Crazy in Alabama	Martial Law	Worst-Case Scenario
Crossing Jordan	Matrix Reloaded	The Young and the Restless
Daredevil	Matrix Revolutions	
Fastlane	Monster-in-Law	

Jennifer Worick is the coauthor of *The Action Heroine's Handbook*, *The Worst-Case Scenario Survival Handbook: College,* and the *New York Times* bestseller *The Worst-Case Scenario Survival Handbook: Dating & Sex.* In addition, she has written *Get Your Dating Game On, Girls Night In, Live with a Man and Love It*, and *Nancy Drew's Guide to Life*. She writes regularly for magazines such as *Cosmopolitan* and *Women's Health*. No longer just content to be an armchair action heroine, she seeks out adventure in Philadelphia.